A Year of Grace

A Year of Grace

365 Reflections for Caregivers

Laraine Bennett

Our Sunday Visitor
200 Noll Plaza
Huntington, IN 46750

20 19 18 17 16 15 14   1 2 3 4 5 6 7 8 9

ISBN: 978-1-61278-726-8 (Inventory No. T1436)
eISBN: 978-1-61278-342-0
LCCN: 2014933122
Cover design: Lindsey Riesen
Cover art: Shutterstock
Interior design: Lindsey Riesen

PRINTED IN THE UNITED STATES OF AMERICA

Table of Contents

Foreword

Capernaum, a bustling fishing village on the northwest shore of the Sea of Galilee, is the home of Peter, Andrew, James, and John. On a single day Jesus teaches in the synagogue, performs exorcisms, cures Simon Peter's mother-in-law, and spends the entire evening healing the sick and driving out demons. "The whole town was gathered at the door" (Mk 1:33).

The pressing of the crowds, the groanings of the sick and possessed, the constant clamoring for his attention — all this must have been exhausting for Jesus in His humanity.

So He rises very early — before dawn — to pray (see Mk 1:35).

Isn't the life of a caregiver like this, too? Your work is profoundly rewarding, yet it can also be exhausting, lonely, humiliating, anxiety-provoking, monotonous, and relentless. This demanding daily work requires prayer time. Saints and spiritual writers often remind us that the busier our lives, the more we need to spend time in prayer.

God is always calling us to himself, drawing us with kindness and "bands of love" (Hos 11:4). But we need to take the time to listen to that still, small voice that speaks to our hearts. Most especially, God speaks to us when we take the time to pray.

This book is for you, the caregiver. You don't have much time for yourself, so the reflections are short. They are meant to inspire, encourage, lighten your spirits, and provide food for thought.

So, take just a few minutes of silence, before the duties of life rush in, to reflect on the presence of God all around and within you. It is the presence of a Father who loves you infinitely more that you can even imagine.

> Yet it was I who taught Ephraim to
> walk,
> who took them in my arms....
> I fostered them like those
> who raise an infant to their
> cheeks;
> I bent down to feed them.
>
> — Hosea 11:3-4

Place yourself like a child in His loving arms, ask for His help, listen to His words of comfort and peace that He brings you through Scripture, through meditating on the mysteries of Christ's life, and through these reflections.

I hope this book might bring you warmth, laughter, a stirring of the heart, a feeling of tenderness for the body of Christ who is present to you in the distressing guise of the sick. I hope you feel inspired and encouraged, renewed and strengthened, to meet your day with love.

Dedication

For my mom, Teje

"Chastised a little, they shall be greatly blessed,
because God tried them and found them worthy of himself."

— Wisdom 3:5

As this book was going to press, my mom passed away, surrounded by her family. It was a Marian feast, and it was as though the Blessed Mother was holding Mom's hand as she entered eternal life, just as my mom had held her rosary beads for so many years. The incapacitating stroke that took nearly everything from her but her laughter and her love for family and nature was also a blessing that brought us together in a wholly different way. I will be forever grateful for the gift and blessing of her life.

"Blessed be the God and Father of our Lord Jesus Christ, the Father of compassion and God of all encouragement, who encourages us in our every affliction, so that we may be able to encourage those who are in any affliction with the encouragement with which we ourselves are encouraged by God."

— 2 Corinthians 1:3-4

January 1

Quiet Within

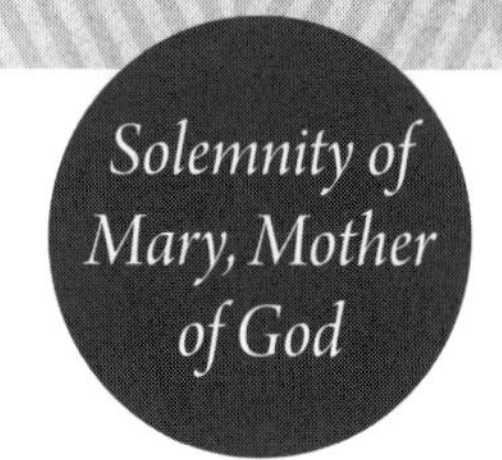

"And Mary kept all these things, reflecting on them in her heart."

— Luke 2:19

My mom was born in Germany and studied at the prestigious Academy of Art in Berlin. Then, she had her appendix removed to get out of working for Hitler's war effort — she called it her "political appendix." She fell in love with an American soldier, and shook the dust of Europe off her feet when she emigrated. Perhaps because of a stormy relationship with her own mother, she embraced the Blessed Mother when she converted to Catholicism. An all-round artist, she loved music, writing, cooking, and painting. Though she could no longer speak or walk, write or eat, much less paint, following her stroke, she — like Mary — kept all these things in her heart.

January 2

The Mystery of Suffering

"When it was evening, after sunset, they brought to him all who were ill or possessed by demons. The whole town was gathered at the door."

— Mark 1:32-33

You can just imagine the scene: an entire city bringing their sick and possessed! People were moaning and crying out, pushing and shoving at the door. And when Jesus heals them, He doesn't do it like the Great and Powerful Oz from behind a curtain or even through a philanthropic foundation, sending money in from afar. Instead, He touches each suffering one, looking in the eyes of each one, acknowledging each one as a person with dignity. He forgives their sins, and sometimes (but not always) cures them physically.

JANUARY 3

Breath Prayer

Feast of the Most Holy Name of Jesus

"Because of this, God greatly exalted him and bestowed on him the name that is above every name, that at the name of Jesus every knee should bend, of those in heaven and on earth and under the earth, and every tongue confess that Jesus Christ is Lord."

— Philippians 2:9-11

There was a monk of Mount Athos who prayed to Mary, the Theotokos, that he might be given the gift of praying without ceasing. He received what is now called the Jesus Prayer, which is prayed even today by Orthodox monks: "*Lord Jesus Christ, Son of the living God, have mercy on me, a sinner.*" The Jesus Prayer is similar to the prayer of the blind Bartimaeus who cried out to Jesus with all his heart and soul for healing.

On those days when you feel all tapped out, dry and empty inside, try saying this "breath prayer," a prayer that can be said with a single breath as the individual inhales and exhales. Feel it lift your soul.

January 4

Where Are You Staying?

"Jesus turned and saw them following him and said to them, 'What are you looking for?' They said to him, 'Rabbi' (which translated means Teacher), 'where are you staying?'"

— John 1:38

John the Baptist was hugely popular and had a following from all over Judea, including the city of Jerusalem. So it's startling when he suddenly stops preaching and says, "Behold, the Lamb of God" (Jn 1:36). Two of his disciples immediately run after the man John is referring to. Jesus turns and says to them, "What are you looking for?" And they answer with a question. That part always puzzles me.

What am I looking for? Lord, there are so many things. I don't know what to say: healing for my mom, direction for me, happiness for my kids. Oh, and my car has 150,000 miles on it! Instead of answering, the disciples ask: "Where are you staying?" Maybe if I just spend time with Him, I will know what I am looking for. I will have the answer I seek.

JANUARY 5

Feeling Empty

"When they walk through the Valley of Weeping, it will become a place of refreshing springs. The autumn rains will clothe it with blessings."

— Psalm 84:6, New Living Translation

There are days, I am sure, when it seems as though you are dragging yourself through that bitter Valley of Weeping. You feel tired, empty, and your love tank seems emptied of all compassion. Even though you may feel dry, God is nonetheless working through you, working through the very emptiness. In fact, these days will count all the more in the eternal kingdom. God is blessing your work, sending His gentle rain upon the dry earth.

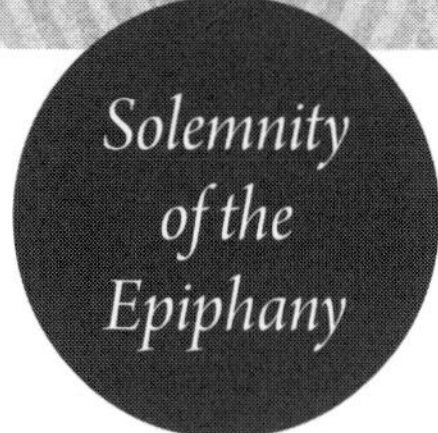

JANUARY 6

Star of Wonder, Star of Light

"To look at the star means receiving light and giving light."

— Cardinal Joseph Ratzinger, *The Blessing of Christmas*

The magi travel from the East, following a star. They are wise men on a search. If they had been astronomers, they could have stayed home and peered through their telescopes. And if astrologers, they would have been satisfied with their myths and occult *woowoo.* But they are truth seekers; so they journey. We, too, are journeying through life seeking truth. In order to find our way, we must follow a star. What — or *who* — is my guiding star?

January 7

A Precious Gift of Self

"And on entering the house they saw the child with Mary his mother. They prostrated themselves and did him homage. Then they opened their treasures and offered him gifts of gold, frankincense, and myrrh."

— Matthew 2:11

As a caregiver, you bring precious treasures to your loved one. Like gold, your smile brings a joy that is worth more than gold. Your encouragement is like the fragrant incense that rises to heaven. And your gentle touch is like the anointing of sacred oil. These are like the treasures the three wise men brought to Jesus. And you are bringing the greatest treasure of all — your presence, your gift of self-giving love.

JANUARY 8

Patiently Waiting

"Now there is in Jerusalem at the Sheep [Gate] a pool called in Hebrew Bethesda, with five porticoes. In these lay a large number of ill, blind, lame, and crippled."

— John 5:2-3

For thirty-eight years, this man has been ill, unable to walk, wanting so desperately to plunge into the healing waters of the pool. You can just picture the scene. As soon as the spirit of God stirs up the water, everyone rushes down to the pool, leaving the poor fellow literally in the dust. The residents of the nursing home wait patiently for someone to come to their room and lift them out of bed. They wait like the man in the Scriptures waited, watching as others get into the water. Waiting for Jesus.

January 9

Grace Breath

"The delicate breath of grace can disperse the blackest clouds, it can make life beautiful and rich with meaning, even in the most inhuman situations."

— Pope Benedict XVI, *Address on the Feast of the Immaculate Conception, at the Spanish Steps, 2012*

We stroll with my mom, pushing her in her wheelchair around the grounds, grateful for the warmth of the sun on our faces. "Got to get that vitamin D!" I enthuse. A delicate breeze blows across the Accotink Trail and through the tall maples, ruffling our hair. Another couple is power walking with their walkers. We take it very slow, squeezing out every drop of fresh air and sunshine. The beauty of nature and the breath of grace free us from the sick bed, the medical equipment, the dependence on nurses.

January 10

Hope

"Why are you downcast, my soul? . . .

Wait for God, for I shall again praise him."

— Psalm 42:6

Irene asks me to look in her orthopedic bootie. "I think there's a letter for me from Barstow, Alaska," she says. I am puzzled. She explains that she has applied for a teaching job there. All her life she has wanted to live in Alaska. "When I get out of here, that's what I want to do." "Here" is a nursing home, and Irene, in her mid-eighties, has suffered an incapacitating stroke. I love her positive attitude, and it makes me think that I should be more hopeful, too.

JANUARY 11

Eagle Wings

"I bore you up on eagles' wings and brought you to myself."

— Exodus 19:4

I had been waiting for several months for a medical flight to open up to bring my mom to Virginia. All the while, I was praying a novena to Saint Joseph. Finally, on Saint Joseph's feast day, we flew out together in a private jet. It was thrilling for me, and a little scary for my mom. Still, the answered prayer (for me) and the flight away from her beloved home into the unknown (for my mom) brings home an important message. God is always calling us to Him, always — though sometimes quite mysteriously — bringing us closer to himself.

January 12

Laughter is the Best Medicine

"'And why the devil that young woman won't sit down like a Christian,' says Mr. George with his eyes musingly fixed on Judy, 'I can't comprehend.'

"'She keeps at my side to attend to me, sir,' says Grandfather Smallweed. 'I am an old man, my dear Mr. George, and I need some attention.'"

— Charles Dickens, *Bleak House*

Grandfather Smallweed continuously slides down in his chair, collapsing in a shapeless bundle. Judy picks him up, shakes him out like an old rag, and repositions him with a poke of the finger. I used to tease my mom that she was like a sack of potatoes or Grandfather Smallweed. But now, sadly, she no longer gets our shared joke. Instead, she will chuckle if I say something clearly outrageous ("Don't stay out late dancing!") or do something silly like jumping jacks at the foot of her bed. I try for all the silliness I can muster, just to get a laugh. Sometimes, a good laugh is truly healing.

January 13

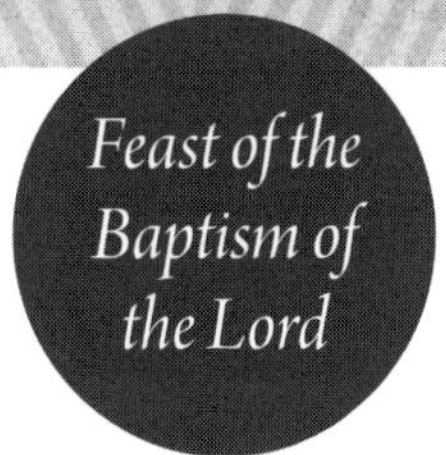

Life-giving Water

"Let the one who thirsts come forward, and the one who wants it receive the gift of life-giving water."

— Revelation 22:17

As Jesus is being baptized by John, the heavens open and the spirit of God descends like a dove. A voice comes from the heavens saying: "This is my beloved Son, with whom I am well pleased" (Mt 3:17). At our first grandchild's baptism, the young deacon sings *Come to the Water* a cappella. We are astounded. This is the very song we played at the baptism of our son — the one whose son is being baptized! God is opening heaven at this moment, and showering His grace on us.

We thirst, and sometimes this thirst is the dryness of our daily routine, the parched feeling of being emotionally drained. We must remember that God merely wants us to step forward and receive His gift, His life-giving water.

January 14

Little Things

"We ought not to be weary of doing little things for the love of God, who regards not the greatness of the work, but the love with which it is performed."

— Brother Lawrence, *The Practice of the Presence of God*

Brother Lawrence of the Resurrection was a humble monk who worked in the monastery kitchen and repaired the sandals of his Carmelite brothers. For a number of years, he struggled with nearly paralyzing anxiety and fear. Then one day, he discovered the answer and was flooded with inner peace in the presence of God. Instead of worrying about the future or dwelling on mistakes of his past, he looked for God in the present moment, cultivating a constant awareness of God within. The key is doing every little thing out of love for God.

January 15

Dogs and Good Samaritans

"Do not neglect hospitality, for through it some have unknowingly entertained angels."

— Hebrews 13:2

Who are these people who give so freely of their time, visiting folks they don't even know? One man brings his Irish wolfhound, Blackie. The dog's head is larger than my grandson and looms, shaggy and docile, over hospital beds. His big nose (the size of a baseball!) gently pokes at my mom's hand. She laughs with delight and exclaims, "Whoa! Whoa!" We love petting this gentle giant. I hope that someday I will be as generous as this man who brings his beloved pet to cheer strangers.

JANUARY 16

The Kingdom of God

"[Jesus] said, 'To what shall we compare the kingdom of God? ... It is like a mustard seed that, when it is sown in the ground, is the smallest of all the seeds on the earth. But once it is sown, it springs up and becomes the largest of plants and puts forth large branches, so that the birds of the sky can dwell in its shade.'"

— Mark 4:30-32

Have you ever seen a mustard seed? It is so tiny and negligible. It looks as though it will never amount to much. Just so, sometimes the daily work of a caregiver seems inconsequential. But like the mustard seed when it springs up, that work creates a place of rest and peace. It could be a gentle massage for the bedridden, a cool towel for one who is in pain, a smile and a greeting for the lonely. The tiny seed becomes the kingdom of God.

January 17

Our Neighbor

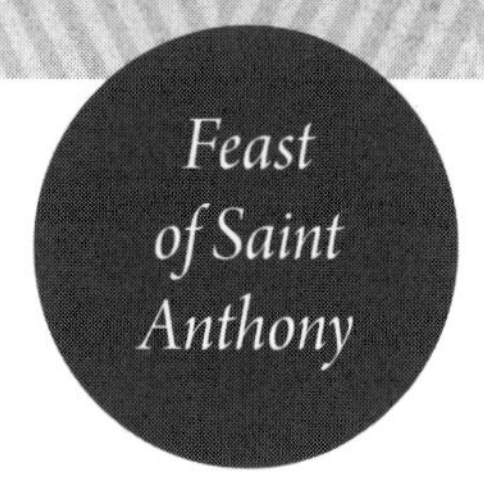

"Abba Antony said, 'Our life and our death are with our neighbor. If we gain our brother, we have gained our God.'"

— *Daily Readings with the Desert Fathers*

When Anthony was a young man, his parents died and left him their estate. He had heard the words of the Gospel about the rich young man who went away sad when Jesus recommended he sell his possessions (see Mt 19:16-22). Anthony vowed to give away everything to the poor, except what his sister needed to live on. Later, he went away to live in the desert, becoming one of the first Christian hermits. He lived at the top of a mountain, working in his little garden, fasting and praying continually. He told his monks that the devil dreads fasting, prayer, humility, and good works. Let us persevere, with Saint Anthony's help, in all of these!

January 18

Looking for Heaven

"I am weary with crying out;

my throat is parched.

My eyes fail,

from looking for my God."

— Psalm 69:4

Just before I enter her room, I see my mom lying in bed, quiet. Her pale blue eyes are looking out the window. Does she long to see another sight? My handsome dad, dressed in his fatigues and combat boots, grinning from ear to ear? Does she long to be young once more, and run into his arms? The sky will be lavender and gold, jasper and carnelian, the glassy sea sparkling in the radiance of the Lamb. And everyone will cheer as they welcome a new saint to eternal life.

JANUARY 19

Burning Bush

"Your relationship with God is unique. He has a mission reserved for you that no other person can accomplish."

— Mother Angelica, *Answers, Not Promises*

On an ordinary day, Moses receives an extraordinary call: to lead the Israelites out of slavery in Egypt. He's tending his sheep when he sees a bush on fire — burning, yet not consumed. Curious, he goes nearer and hears the voice of God.

On an ordinary day, we might hear the voice of God speaking to our hearts. Do we draw nearer so we can listen? And then, do we, like Moses, make many objections? Who am I that I should go to Egypt? Who will I say is telling me to do this? What if they don't believe me? And besides, I am slow of speech! God assures him, just as He assures us, "*I will be with you!*"

January 20

Rich in What Matters

"Thus it will be for the one who stores up treasure for himself but is not rich in what matters to God."

— Luke 12:21

We pack the moving van like a Chinese puzzle, furniture and boxes stacked high and wedged in to maximize our space. I wonder whether I will need to rent a storage unit to keep all the furniture and mementos from my parents' home. This reminds me of the parable of the rich man who decides to build larger barns for all his grain and his goods. He wants to retire without worries, eat, drink, and be merry. God says: "You fool, this night your life will be demanded of you" (Lk 12:20). Jesus explains that this is how it will be, for those who are not rich in what matters to God.

But if you who care for others with love, you are rich in what matters.

January 21

Oil of Gladness

"He has sent me to bring good news to the afflicted,

to bind up the brokenhearted,

To proclaim liberty to the captives."

— Isaiah 61:1

Who is more captive than those confined to beds, whether at home or in nursing homes? They may be unable to move, unable to speak, helpless, utterly dependent on the attention of their caregivers. The prophet in the Book of Isaiah says that the Lord will give them "oil of gladness" and a "glorious mantle" instead of a listless spirit.

I visit the nursing home every day now. How I wish I could bring the residents this oil of gladness, this glorious mantle. Instead, I greet them with a cheery "Hello! How's it going?" My cousin Ruth knits a glorious cashmere shawl for my mom. I flag down the priest with the yellow Jeep Wrangler, and he anoints my mom's forehead with sacred oil. We do what we can do!

January 22

Seats of Honor

"He has scattered the proud in the imagination of their hearts, he has put down the mighty from their thrones, and exalted those of low degree."

— Luke 1:51, RSVCE

The Pharisees love being seated at places of honor at banquets and Jesus denounces them: "Whoever exalts himself will be humbled" (Mt 23:12). At the nursing home, the residents are wheeled out to the dining area where they wait patiently for someone to bring them their meals. They wait for someone to hold a spoon to their lips, bring them a glass of water. Jesus tells them: "You will be exalted."

JANUARY 23

A Precious Life

"However difficult or however insignificant our life may seem to be, it is precious to God as Christ is precious to God."

— Caryll Houselander, *The Passion of the Infant Christ*

A Canadian woman with a degenerative brain disease decides that her best option is to leave her home, family, and friends, and fly to Switzerland, where she can legally commit suicide. She is only seventy-two. She says good-bye to her family at the airport, tears streaming down her face. Her grandchildren are clinging to her and crying, confused. Why is Grandma leaving? She could allow the disease to progress and eventually die at home several years hence, surrounded by loved ones. Or she can take matters into her own hands, fly to Switzerland, drink poison, and die alone. Let us pray that this poor soul finds peace.

January 24

Feast of Saint Francis de Sales

Called to Holiness

"Through devotion your family cares become more peaceful, mutual love between husband and wife becomes more sincere... and our work, no matter what it is, becomes more pleasant and agreeable."

— Saint Francis de Sales, *Introduction to the Devout Life*

Saint Francis teaches us that each one of us, no matter our position in life — whether old or young, married or single, poor or rich — is called to holiness. Yes, holiness, as in Saint Britney, Saint Dylan, Saint Fill-in-the-Blank! Holiness is not just for priests and religious; it's for each one of us. Moreover, this holiness doesn't turn us into censorious sourpusses. Rather, it makes us happy, peaceful, and loving.

Conversion of Saint Paul the Apostle

January 25

Light Dawns

"Now I want you to know, brothers, that the gospel preached by me is not of human origin. For I did not receive it of a human being, nor was I taught it, but it came through a revelation of Jesus Christ."

— Galatians 1:11

Caravaggio's dramatic painting shows Paul's moment of conversion: flat on his back, horse with hoof raised above him. Other Caravaggio paintings capture action, but here all is stillness: the horse in mid-step, the sword dropped, Saul's eyes closed against the blinding light. We imagine Christ's voice, though He is not pictured here: "Why are you persecuting me?" (see Acts 9:1-9). Sometimes Jesus lets us know exactly how our actions hurt — or console — Him.

January 26

Opening the Gates

"Gate of heaven, teach our hearts to desire the things of heaven."

— Saint John XXIII, *Prayers and Devotions*

Mary's daughter, Courtney, has suffered grand mal seizures daily for the past twenty years. She is unable to walk or talk and can see only shadows. But she hums and laughs, loves music and listening to her brother read to her. Her mother says she has one foot in heaven and one firmly planted on earth. Doctors don't know what causes the seizures, and they never expected her to live beyond three years of age. Today, and every day, Courtney's mom tells her, "I kiss the hands that have opened for me the gates of heaven."

JANUARY 27

Handing Over the Burden

"Carrying one another's burdens is not just a figure of speech or something meaningful only in terms of physical burdens like a trunk. Davy's burden was not death but the fear of death. I asked her to give me that burden, a real handing over, like surrendering a trunk to a porter. An act of handing over. And I took it — also act. I then entered into the fear, her fear, with all my heart and mind and imagination, felt it, carried it along with my own fear, which was also real but other. And her burden grew lighter."

— Sheldon Vanauken, *A Severe Mercy*

We should consciously seek to share one another's burden. Ask them to hand it over.

January 28

A Youthful Soul

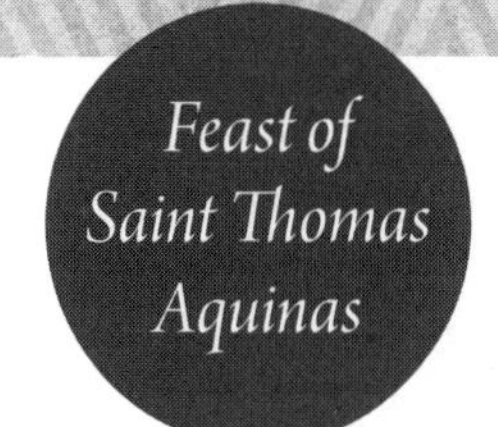

"Grant me, O Lord my God, a mind to know you, a heart to seek you, wisdom to find you, conduct pleasing to you, faithful perseverance in waiting for you, and a hope of finally embracing you."

— Prayer of Saint Thomas Aquinas

After her first stroke (but before the most recent, calamitous one) my mom would say, "Getting old is the pits!" I asked her once: "How old do you *feel*, inside?" She said, about thirty. Thirty-three is the perfect age, according to Saint Thomas Aquinas. It's the age we'll be in heaven, the age Jesus chose to suffer and die on the Cross, the height of our physical powers. It's the age of our souls all the time, no matter how our bones ache, our arthritis bothers us, or our hearing or memory fails. Our souls are eternally young.

January 29

Our True Home

"My dwelling, like a shepherd's tent,

is struck down and borne away from me;

You have folded up my life, like a weaver

who severs me from the last thread."

— Isaiah 38:12

The anguished cries of the mortally ill Hezekiah are answered by God, who gives him a miraculous sign of His healing: the shadow of the sun retreats ten steps. Indeed, God can sever the last thread, strike down the tent. My mom's house is only now paid off, in the same year that she is literally struck down. The massive stroke means she will never again dwell in her home. We pray for healing, as did King Hezekiah. Still, her true home comes every day nearer, advancing like the sun on the steps of Ahaz.

JANUARY 30

Holy Stairs, Precious Blood

"O Jesus, when I consider the great price of Your Blood, I rejoice at its immensity, for one drop alone would have been enough for the salvation of all sinners."

— Saint Faustina, *Diary*

The *Scala Sancta*, the Holy Stairs, which once led to Pilate's praetorium in Jerusalem, were brought to Rome by Saint Helena. We climb the stairs on our knees, the wood polished smooth and indented from thousands of faithful pilgrims' knees. Do I see a drop of blood, saving blood from Jesus' passion, on the marble beneath the wood? Caring for a loved one is like wiping a drop of blood from Our Lord's brow.

January 31

The Measure

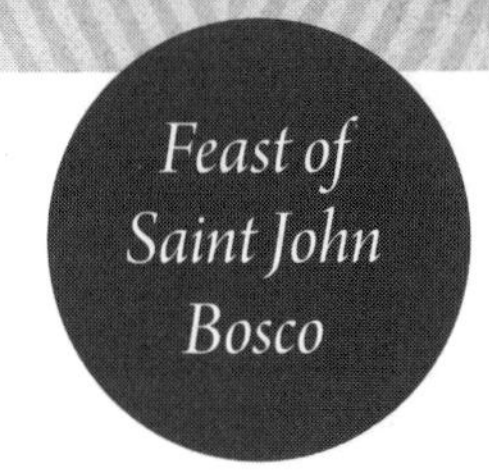

"You should bear patiently the bad temper of other people, the slights, the rudeness that may be offered you."

— Saint John Bosco, *Quotable Saints*

When we think about the scourging, the thorns digging into His skull, the jeers and mockery that Christ bore during His Passion, we shouldn't be so resentful when someone is merely rude to us. Yet, so often I respond with harsh words or scathing looks when someone dares to cross me. When old Mrs. X. whines, "Your mother doesn't like your hair like that," I am indignant, as though she could even help it. Then, I remember that Jesus said, "The measure with which you measure will be measured out to you" (Mk 4:24).

I resolve to respond with gentleness and compassion, no matter how I feel.

FEBRUARY 1

Living Stones

"Abbot Pastor said . . . If there are three monks living together, of whom one remains silent in prayer at all times, and another is ailing and gives thanks for it, and the third waits on them both with sincere good will, these three are equal, as if they were performing the same work."

— Thomas Merton, *The Wisdom of the Desert*

The caregiver and the one who is cared for: both are a living prayer.

February 2

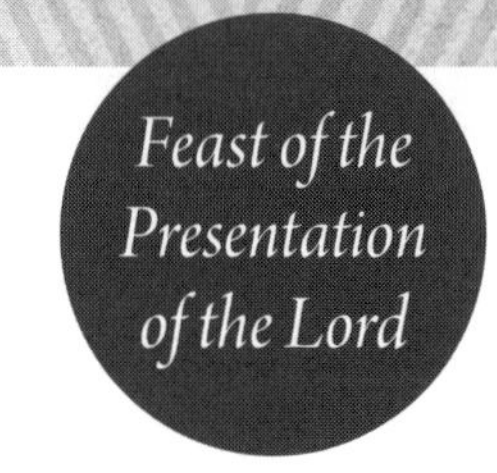

Dispelling Darkness

"'Now, Master, you may let your servant go in peace, according to your word, for my eyes have seen your salvation.'"

— Luke 2:29-30

Simeon was an old man, devout and righteous, prayerful. The Holy Spirit revealed to him that he would not die before seeing the Lord. Is he surprised when the Lord comes to him as a baby? Filled with the spirit, he is at the Temple that very day, taking the baby in his arms and praising God. We bring our first grandchild to my mom. Both he and she laugh, and coo and smile.

This day, we *present* our loved ones to God, and ask Him to bless us, to shine His light on us, and to dispel our darkness.

February 3

Climbing to Heaven

"Who may go up the mountain of the Lord?

Who can stand in his holy place?

The clean of hand and pure of heart."

— Psalm 24:3-4

Old Rag Mountain has an elevation over three thousand feet. The hike to the summit is strenuous at times, with a mile-long rock scramble. The views from the top are spectacular. The Blue Ridge Mountains, true to their name, rise like oceanic waves atop a lush, green, tree canopy. I wouldn't be able to make it without a hand from above and a push from behind. Climbing God's mountain is like that, too. We need God's grace, and we need the saints in heaven praying us forward, and our friends pushing us from behind.

February 4

Serving God

"Whatever, wherever I am, I can never be thrown away. If I am in sickness, my sickness may serve Him; in perplexity, my perplexity may serve Him; if I am in sorrow, my sorrow may serve Him."

— Blessed John Henry Newman

We are always part of God's plan. Even at our most destitute, downtrodden, and helpless, we are important to God. He loves us. He wants us to accomplish a mission, even if it *seems* very small and insignificant. Even if we are not aware of it.

February 5

Whatsoever You Do

"I wake and feel the fell of dark, not day.

What hours, O what black hours we have spent

This night! What sights you, heart, saw; ways you went!

And more must, in yet longer light's delay."

— Gerard Manley Hopkins, *I Wake and Feel*

When I stayed with my mom in her home, I would awaken in the middle of the night, hearing her walker clunking and scraping its way to the bathroom. My ears would strain, I would hold my breath, hoping she would make it safely back to bed. Then I would peek into her room and wish her sweet dreams. I always sensed that Jesus whispered back, "Thank you."

February 6

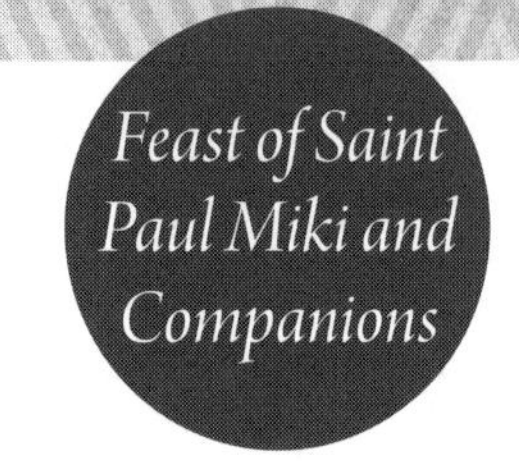

Martyrdom

"For it has been granted to you that for the sake of Christ you should not only believe in him but also suffer for his sake."

— Philippians 1:29, RSVCE

Paul Miki, a Japanese Jesuit novice, was imprisoned along with other Catholics when the emperor became fearful of their influence. Miki and twenty-five companions were forced to march 600 miles from Kyoto to Nagasaki where they were crucified on February 5, 1597. He preached his last sermon from the cross, forgiving his executioners. This makes our daily trials seem much lighter.

FEBRUARY 7

Remembering the Good Things

"I turned every way, but there was no one to help; I looked for support but there was none. Then I remembered the mercies of the LORD, his acts of kindness through ages past."

— Ben Sira (Sirach) 51:7-8

The Book of Sirach (called the Wisdom of Ben Sira in the revised edition of the New American Bible) is a collection of wise sayings or maxims. The author reminds us that during those times when it seems that you have no one to help or support you, when you are bearing the burden of caregiving all alone, remember the ways God has helped you in the past. This is wise, indeed! Researchers on the science of happiness tell us that remembering (or better, keeping a daily journal about) the things we are grateful for — even the smallest things — will make us happier people.

Remember God's mercy, and call upon Him now. He will not abandon you.

February 8

People or Possessions?

"All these toys were never intended to possess my heart . . . my true good is in another world and my only real treasure is Christ."

— C.S. Lewis, *The Problem of Pain*

After God forgives the Ninevites (see Jon 3:10), Jonah builds himself a little hut and sits in the sun, sulking. God sends a kikayon plant to give him shade. When the plant withers and dies, Jonah tells God that he would be better off dead. How easily we become attached to our possessions! The more we have, the greater our anxiety and the more we need. God asks Jonah: What is more important, people or possessions?

When you are caring for another person, you have the better part!

February 9

Simplicity of Love

"There is a balm in Gilead to make the wounded whole;

There is a balm in Gilead to heal the sin-sick soul."

— Traditional Spiritual

Henri Nouwen, who lived and worked with L'Arche, a community of caregivers, writes that he was once struggling to help friends solve marriage difficulties. He suddenly had an insight: instead of trying to *solve* their problems, he should be an instrument of God's healing. Sometimes, we try so hard to solve problems and to be helpful that it all becomes burdensome. Perhaps we should realize the greater value of simply carrying God's healing message of love.

February 10

When the Job Is Overwhelming

"I will not leave you desolate; I will come to you."

— John 14:18, RSVCE

When Cardinal Joseph Ratzinger was elected pope, he didn't want the job. This thoughtful, quiet man had hoped to retire, live with his brother in a small Bavarian village, play the piano, and write. Instead, he was thrust onto the world stage to bear the burden of leading the entire Church. He tells us that at that very moment: "The words that resounded in my heart were: 'Lord, what do you ask of me? It is a great weight that you are placing on my shoulders but, if you ask it of me, I will cast my nets at your command, confident that you will guide me, even with all my weaknesses.'"

Caregivers, too, often feel their burden deeply. But cast yourself on God's mercy and He will help you.

February 11

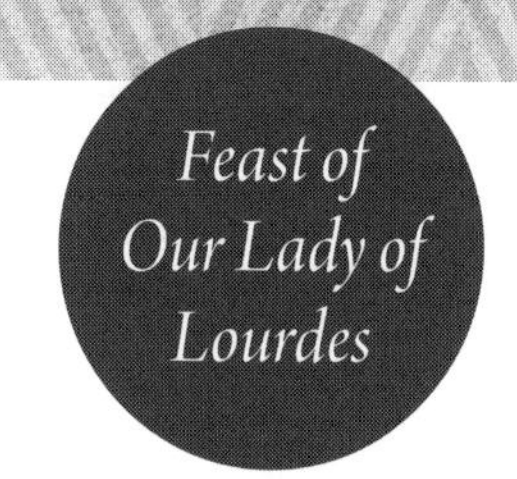

Lourdes, Everywhere!

"I realize that I need not be at Lourdes to find peace and joy. Lourdes simply reminds me that purity, simplicity, and freedom belong to the heart and can be lived anywhere."

— Henri Nouwen, *Mornings with Henri Nouwen*

I know a priest who was cured of cancer after visiting Lourdes. But more important, his heart was cured of its worldly desires. Most of us will never visit Lourdes, nor can we take our sick loved ones. But, we can visit Lourdes in our hearts by remaining close to our Blessed Mother. She will bring us to Christ, just as she did when visiting Elizabeth while carrying Jesus in her womb. And she will help us remain with Him, just as she remained at the foot of the Cross.

February 12

Humility

"They began to salute him with, 'Hail, King of the Jews!' and kept striking his head with a reed and spitting upon him."

— Mark 15:18-19

After the Roman soldiers had scourged and mocked Him, Jesus was stripped of His clothes and given the Cross. What a contrast to the gentle bathing and changing and dressing that caregivers provide! Still, it is a true cross for the one who no longer can do anything for himself or herself. Let us pray for the grace to humbly accept both care and caregiving!

February 13

Stories

"When we put our elders in nursing homes with a couple of mothballs in their pockets as if they were an overcoat, in a certain sense our nostalgic side has failed us, since being with our grandparents means coming face-to-face with our past."

— Pope Francis, *Conversations with Jorge Bergoglio: His Life in His Own Words:*

We look at family photographs from the 1940s. There are black-and-white photos of my dad riding a horse on his sister's ranch. There are other photos of my dad's brothers and sisters (all but one now dead) in the Basque hotel where they grew up. There's even one of my grandfather castrating a sheep the "humane" way — with his teeth. (Google it; it's not as far-fetched as it sounds!) My mom recognizes these people, but she is no longer able to tell me more.

Scripture has it: "Remember the days of old, consider the years of generations past. Ask your father, he will inform you, your elders, they will tell you" (Dt 32:7). If you are caring for an older relative or parent, ask for their stories.

February 14

Believe in Love

Feast of Saints Cyril and Methodius; Saint Valentine's Day

"When you hear all sorts of things announced by this leader or that, but no mention of love, be on your guard, my children, beware."

— Saint John XXIII, *Prayers and Devotions*

Saint Valentine has long been honored on this day although observance of his feast was officially dropped from the liturgical calendar in 1969. We can continue to honor Saint Valentine, but today we also venerate Saints Cyril and Methodius who were missionaries in Slavic lands. All three gave their lives for Christ

Since it's Valentine's Day, it seems appropriate to mention that he was a saint who believed in love. He secretly married young lovers who were being forced to remain unwed because of the emperor's demand for single men in the Roman military. Today, in the spirit of Saint Valentine, let's show everyone that we believe in love.

February 15

Burden of Caregiving

"It would be naive to ignore the suffering and discouragement, the sadness and loneliness that meet us relentlessly as we go through life. But our faith has taught us with absolute certainty . . . that everything around and in us is impregnated with divine purpose, that all things echo the call beckoning us to the house of our Father."

— Saint Josemaría Escrivá, *Christ Is Passing By*

Moses leads his people out of slavery and through the desert on the way to the Promised Land. He feeds them, cares for them, and prays for them. Yet all they do is grumble and complain. When God sends them miraculous manna, they moan that they have no meat. Moses is so fed up that he begs God: "I cannot carry all this people by myself, for they are too heavy for me. If this is the way you will deal with me, then please do me the favor of killing me at once" (Nm 11:14-15).

Even the great prophet Moses, at times, felt so overwhelmed by the burden of caregiving that he wanted to die. Sometimes, we have to be honest with God and tell Him we have reached the breaking point.

February 16

Doctors and Nurses

"To be truly wise is to have learned to see God, but to see God is also to see and love and labor for the world he has made."

— Gerald Vann, O.P., *Heart of Compassion*

Doctor Kelly calls to tell me that my mom's saline levels are way too high. Her kidneys are in distress. We can admit her to the hospital, which will be stressful for her, or we can administer an IV solution right here. I choose the IV solution right here. Sounds like a no-brainer. But then he adds, "I don't know *why* her levels are high; they could figure that out in the hospital."

He wants me to decide. I'm growing anxious. The stress could make her situation worse. I run to talk to the nurses. They tell me not to worry, saying that Doctor Kelly always looks on the gloomy side. We decide to keep my mom in her bed, and within a day, her levels are back to normal. The doctor gives me a hug. What a blessing — these nurses and doctors!

February 17

Revived

"To still waters he leads me;

he restores my soul."

— Psalm 23:2-3

Mrs. X. is whining from her wheelchair, "Can anybody get me a cup of water?" The nursing assistants are studiously avoiding Mrs. X. So, I go to the water cooler and get a cup for her. The assistant whispers, "She won't like it, and she'll yell at you." This reminds me of the woman at the well, who thought she needed water but instead discovers grace. Only the living water of Christ, the water of truth, will truly refresh us and restore our soul. It will soothe our drooping spirits.

February 18

Transformation of the Body

"So also is the resurrection of the dead. . . . It is sown weak; it is raised powerful. It is sown a natural body; it is raised a spiritual body."

— 1 Corinthians 15:42-44

In our vegetable garden we grow arugula and other lettuces from seed. The tasty peppery plant that pops up from its burial ground is completely different from the tiny seed that was planted. Saint Paul shows us that what is true in nature is surely true in super-nature! As our bodies become more and more frail and decrepit, as we are slouching toward death, why doubt that in the next life we will be gloriously transformed and resplendent?

February 19

Laying on Hands

"They will pick up snakes in their hands, and if they drink any deadly thing, it will not harm them; they will lay their hands on the sick, and they will recover."

— Mark 16:18, NRSVCE

My hands do not perform this kind of healing. I massage coconut-lime scented lotion on my mom's hands and arms, and she cries out in pain. "What is it?" I ask. "Are you hurt?" I am alarmed and fetch the nurse. Naphtali, one of the best nurses, comes in immediately and soothes my mom, checking her hand and wrist. There's nothing wrong! "Touch my arm," Naphtali tells me. "Your hands are cold!" he laughs. Then all three of us burst out laughing!

February 20

Releasing Control

"For surely I know the plans I have for you, says the LORD, plans for your welfare, not for harm."

— Jeremiah 29:11, NRSVCE

How often we think we are in control of everything about our lives. We make our plans, we determine our direction. Yet we don't really understand who we are, much less our purpose! "Lord, you have probed me, you know me. . . . You understand my thoughts from afar" (Ps 139:1-2).

When I worry about how we can save money, or what I should do about the car, or whether I should sell my parents' house, I become anxious and worried. But, God knows *all of this*, and He wants me to place *all of this* in His hands. He knows what is best for me, for us.

February 21

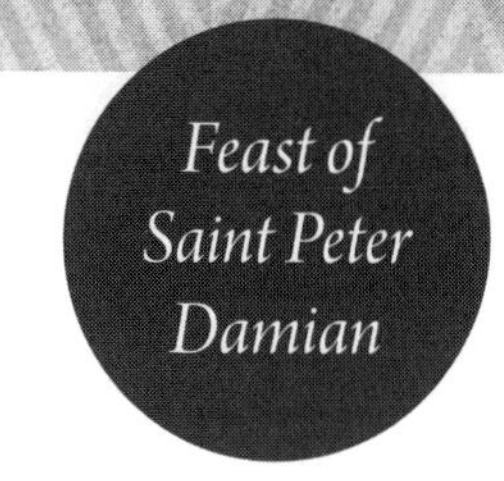

Consolation is Within Reach

"Do not be depressed. Do not let your weakness make you impatient. Instead, let the serenity of your spirit shine through your face."

— Saint Peter Damien

A friend of Saint Peter Damian wrote to him, asking for some words of consolation, as he was undergoing many trials and was feeling depressed and bitter. Peter wrote back: "You don't need my words; consolation is already within your reach!" All our humiliations, sufferings, and tribulations will prove us worthy. Tested, we will shine. This very moment, consolation is within our reach!

February 22

Rock of Faith

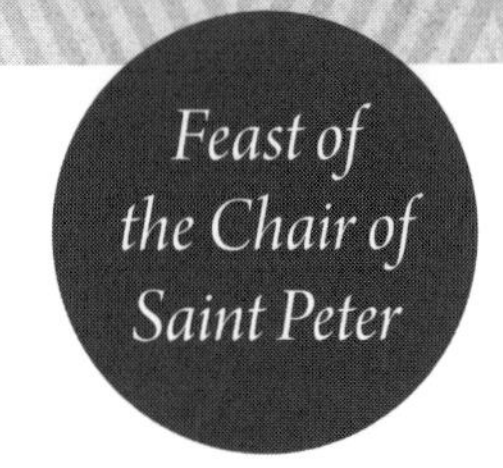

"On this rock I will build my church, and the gates of Hades shall not prevail against it."

— Matthew 16:18, NRSVCE

Instead of a saint's feast day, today we celebrate the Chair of Saint Peter. This chair represents the authority that Christ himself gives to the pope: "On this rock [the rock that is Peter] I will build my church." Sometimes, the nurses and their assistants are so tired, yet they cannot sit down. We put our trust in them, they are our rock. And our rock is our faith, too. Without trust our lives would be as shifting sands, unmoored, despairing.

FEBRUARY 23

Prayer, the Super-Power

"[Prayer's] only art is to call back the souls of the dead from the very journey into death, to give strength to the weak, to heal the sick, to exorcise the possessed, to open prison cells, to free the innocent from their chains."

— Tertullian, *Treatise on Prayer*

In the fiery furnace that was heated seven times stronger than it had ever been, prayer saved Shadrach, Mesach, and Abednego from death (see Dn 3:19-94). My daily prayer may save me from worry, fear, and the flames of anger.

February 24

Connectedness

"I was suddenly overwhelmed with the realization that I loved all those people, that they were mine and I theirs, that we could not be alien to one another even though we were total strangers."

— Thomas Merton, *Confessions*

Thomas Merton had a vision one day while standing on the corner of Fourth and Walnut in downtown Louisville, Kentucky. He describes it as waking from a dream, a dream in which we are all separate and isolated individuals. He discovers that we are really all connected. And each one is shining like the sun. If we think about how God himself became one of us, then we might see those whom we care for shining like the sun.

FEBRUARY 25

A Living Sacrifice

"Offer your bodies as a living sacrifice, holy and pleasing to God, your spiritual worship."

— Romans 12:1

You are caring for your neighbor, whether it is a friend or beloved relative. You are a Good Samaritan, caring for the least of God's children. You are offering your body as a living sacrifice — lifting helpless bodies, feeding and changing, bathing, answering every cry for help.

You are a living sacrifice, holy and acceptable.

February 26

The Last Enemy

"I consider that the sufferings of this present time are as nothing compared to the glory to be revealed for us."

— Romans 8:18

Sometimes, we experience the supernatural mingling with the natural. The hand of God reaches from eternity into time and space, touching us directly. Or, we sense the whispering rustle of evil, like dry leaves swirling behind us on a dark street. Bodily death, our catechism tells us, is the last enemy we must conquer.

As I sit in the hospital room, my mom is hooked up to machines and breathing painfully. The nurse asks about her end-of-life wishes. I know what her wishes are. She wants to be in heaven with her beloved husband of sixty-four years. But God hasn't willed this. She has a battle yet to fight against the enemy that wants to take her soul. I hold her hand. I will help her in this fight.

February 27

Becoming Human

"To live is to love, to think, to suffer; to give oneself; to make out of everything — joys, desires, affections, and griefs — a kind of sublime poem."

— Elizabeth Leseur, *My Spirit Rejoices*

In his homily today, our pastor tells us that we should not try to avoid the Cross, because it is the Cross that makes us truly human. Through the Cross, we learn to love. Jesus says we must take up our cross *daily* (see Lk 9:23). This may mean doing the unpleasant thing, rather than the pleasant. Loving the difficult personality, visiting the shut-in, caring for the sick.

February 28

Working on Faith

"Awake! Why do you sleep, O LORD?"

— Psalm 44:24

This question is answered by Jesus himself, who wakes from His slumber in the boat to calm the winds and the sea. He chastises His friends. "Why are you terrified? Do you not yet have faith?" (see Mk 4:38-40)

How often we are just like the disciples. Despite having walked with Jesus for three or even thirty years, we forget that He is God! We moan and wail: "Don't you *care* that I am drowning here?" Jesus knows that faith is a process: "Do you *not yet* have faith?" This means we have to work at it. Little by little, trial by trial, prayer by prayer, we inch our way forward in faith.

FEBRUARY 29

Living Mindfully

"Pay attention and come to me;

listen, that you may have life."

— Isaiah 55:3

It's Ash Wednesday and I'm listening to National Public Radio as I drive home in stop-and-go traffic. The reporter tells us about an outreach by the Episcopal Church: Ashes to Go! Episcopalian ministers stand around Metro stops and on street corners, distributing ashes.

Ash Wednesday reminds us of our mortality, the tenuous nature of our lives, and it calls us to mindful living. *Mindful living, what a great concept!* I hunt around the car for a scrap of paper and a pen, so I can write it down. *WHAM!* At this very moment, I rear-end the truck in front of me. The lesson is driven home.

March 1

Washing the Feet

"The correct ascent of man occurs precisely where he learns, in humbly turning towards his neighbor, to bow very deeply, down to his feet, down to the gesture of the washing of feet."

— Cardinal Joseph Ratzinger, *Images of Hope*

As a bishop and cardinal in Buenos Aires, Argentina, Jorge Bergoglio washed the feet of AIDs patients. As pope he has washed the feet of prisoners in Rome. Pope Francis has a genuine and long-standing love for the poor and the despised of the world. In Buenos Aires (as in Rome), he refused the official residence and chose to live in a simple apartment, caring for an elderly Jesuit he invited to join him. As Jesus said, "If I . . . the master and teacher, have washed your feet, you ought to wash one another's feet" (Jn 13:14). As a caregiver, you are carrying out Christ's command; in bowing deeply, you will be raised up.

March 2

Mercy

"Blessed are the merciful, for they will be shown mercy."

— Matthew 5:7

Thomas Aquinas wrote that mercy belongs to the nature of God. When we are merciful — when we hold that cup of water to dry lips, answer the cry for help, bring a smile and a sense of humor to the bedridden, or forgive someone for past wrongs — we are being godlike.

MARCH 3

The Bed-Cross

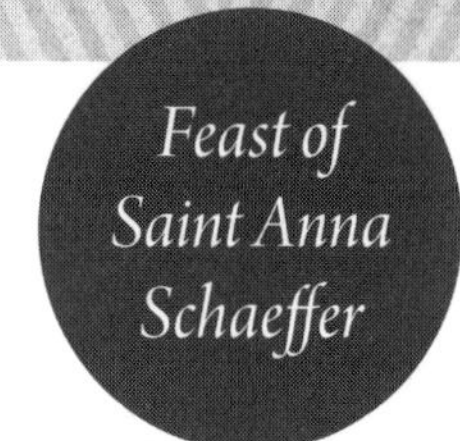

"My life is fading away little by little in suffering. . . . Eternity is ever approaching. Soon, I will live from God, who is Life itself. Heaven has no price, and I rejoice every minute in the Lord's call to the infinitely beautiful homeland."

— Saint Anna Schaeffer

Anna Schaeffer is a beautiful saint both for caregivers and for those who are in need of caregiving. In 1901, not quite nineteen years old, she was working in a laundry and fell into a vat of boiling lye. Her legs were so badly burned that she became an invalid for the rest of her life. Her dreams of becoming a nun were shattered, but she dedicated the rest of her life to praying for others. She called it her "bed-Cross" and offered her suffering in reparation for sins. Though she was weak and never left her bed, she became a saint.

We, too, can offer to God our simple tasks, whatever we might suffer each day, and pray for those who suffer their own bed-Cross.

MARCH 4

Supernatural Entanglement

"In the innermost recesses of existence, there really is such a thing as taking another's place."

— Cardinal Joseph Ratzinger, *Images of Hope*

Quantum theory describes a remarkable phenomenon called entanglement. Particles become permanently correlated, dependent on each other's states and properties, something Albert Einstein called "spooky action at a distance." Maybe this is what ancient religions understood by sacrifice — influencing the gods through their appeasing actions. God goes even further. He sends His only Son as the ultimate and perfect sacrifice. Even our own daily struggles, no matter how small, can be offered for someone else's sake.

March 5

Loving the Imperfect

"My treasures are those souls you have linked with mine."

— Saint Thérèse of Lisieux, *The Story of a Soul*

Saint Thérèse, the Little Flower, wrote that the holiest nuns were the most loved. Everyone wanted to be with them and do things for them. So, she resolved to seek the company of the imperfect, cranky, unfriendly souls and be like the Good Samaritan to them.

The nurses and caregivers at the nursing home are Good Samaritans each and every day. They are surrounded by rejected souls, helpless souls, and all the ones who cannot speak or do for themselves. God will bless and reward this sacrifice!

March 6

A Comforting Mystery

"This Mystery should set before our eyes a vast vision of poor suffering souls: orphans, old people, the sick, the weak, prisoners and exiles. We pray for strength for all these, and the consolation which alone brings hope."

— Saint John XXIII, *Prayers and Devotions*

Christ's life is a mystery. Scripture tells us that when He healed the sick and drove out demons, He "took away our infirmities and bore our diseases" (Mt 8:17). Notice that Jesus doesn't use a magic wand or utter an incantation to make sickness and disease disappear. Rather, He takes them on *himself*. He bears our suffering. This is a *comforting* mystery.

March 7

The Suffering Face of Jesus

"Those tears which spring from the heart of Christ within you are redemptive."

— Gerald Vann, O.P., *Heart of Compassion*

My mom smiles when I wash her face with a warm washcloth. During the sixth Station of the Cross, we focus on Veronica wiping the face of Jesus. We pray: "My beloved Jesus, Your face was beautiful before you began this journey; but, now, it no longer appears beautiful and is disfigured with wounds and blood."

Caregivers wipe the suffering face of Jesus every day. And Christ imprints His face upon their souls.

MARCH 8

Humble Service

Feast of Saint John of God

"Whenever I see so many poor brothers and neighbors of mine suffering beyond their strength and overwhelmed with so many physical or mental ills which I cannot alleviate, then I become exceedingly sorrowful; but I trust in Christ, who knows my heart."

— Saint John of God

There is a faith healer in Brazil who calls himself John of God and claims he channels King Solomon and other figures from the past. Oprah reported his supposedly miraculous healings. The real Saint John of God didn't perform miracles for show. Instead, he humbly served the sick and the poor, bringing blankets to the homeless who lived under bridges, and dressing the wounds of those in his care. He was reviled when he opened homes for prostitutes and the homeless. He was sheltering the worst sorts of people, he was told. But he persevered, eventually founding a religious order, known as the Brother Hospitallers of St. John of God. It is still serving the poor in more than forty countries.

Saint John of God, pray for us!

Feast of Saint Frances of Rome

MARCH 9

Do You Want to Be a Saint?

"Do you really want to be a saint? Carry out the little duty of each moment: do what you ought and concentrate on what you are doing."

— Saint Josemaría Escrivá, *The Way*

We sometimes think the only way to become holy is to die a martyr's death, or to become a pious religious, continually prostrate in front of the altar. Saint Frances of Rome was a strong-willed, resourceful woman who managed a household, and was a dedicated wife and mother. She understood how holiness might come by way of ordinary life. She was devout and prayerful even in the midst of her daily duties as a wife and mother. With her sister-in-law, she ministered to many victims of disease and starvation, even when her own home had been ransacked and nearly destroyed in the Italian civil wars. Eventually, after gaining the blessing of her husband (whom she tenderly cared for), she founded a society of lay women who dedicated themselves to God and to serving the poor. I, too, can strive for holiness while doing my daily duties.

March 10

Constancy

"Standing by the cross of Jesus were his mother and his mother's sister, Mary the wife of Clopas, and Mary of Magdala."

— John 19:25

On Calvary, there are three women at the foot of the Cross, and only one man. The three Marys show us constancy and perseverance in the midst of sorrow and pain. These women show us how love strengthened by sorrow becomes joy. "You will grieve," Jesus tells us, "but your grief will become joy" (Jn 16:20). This helps us bear our present sorrows.

March 11

All Shall Be Well

"All shall be well, all shall be well, and all manner of thing shall be well."

— Julian of Norwich

Little is known about Julian of Norwich other than that she was an anchoress. We don't even know her real name. She prayed that before she was thirty years old she would experience the suffering of Jesus in His Passion, up to the point of His death. And she did. She recovered and wrote down her visions. Her works may be the first written by a woman in English. Out of great suffering (and hiddenness) come beauty and hope for the rest of the world.

March 12

Fiery Chariot

"Sometimes I'm up, and sometimes I'm down,

(Coming for to carry me home)

But still my soul feels heavenly bound.

(Coming for to carry me home)."

— *Swing Low, Sweet Chariot*, hymn

The prophet Elijah never died. Instead, he was taken to heaven in a fiery chariot with flaming horses. I am searching Craigslist for a reclining wheelchair, and I see an ad for a Quickie IRIS Tilt Wheelchair, the Rolls Royce of wheelchairs! I am on the search for whatever it takes to improve my mom's quality of life. I don't want to forget for a moment the value of her time here on earth.

We sometimes get into a rut of "waiting." Waiting for healing, waiting for better times. As though our every moment, no matter how painful or dull or seemingly empty, is not *steeped* in value. And sometimes it takes a fiery chariot (or even a Quickie IRIS) to send our hearts aloft.

March 13

A Difficult Thought

"You have died for love of me; I will die for love of you."

— Saint Alphonsus Liguori, *Stations of the Cross*

When we pray the Stations of the Cross on Fridays during Lent, we say "I accept in particular the death that is destined for me, with all the pains that may accompany it." This is a very difficult thought to grasp! We like to think God chooses for us a particular mission, a vocation, even a spouse. But, does He choose our death, too? We must pray for the grace to accept it.

March 14

Tiny Shoots

And for all this, nature is never spent;

There lives the dearest freshness deep down things."

— Gerard Manley Hopkins, *God's Grandeur*

My cousin brings us a pot of dirt in which paperwhite bulbs are buried. Each day, the tiny green shoots grow a bit taller and we marvel. Caregivers know that it's sometimes the smallest things that can make your heart light, make you sing, revive hope. Courtney's humming, my mom's laughing bright blue eyes, a tiny green shoot poking up out of the dirt, a bird outside the window. God sends us small signs of grace. It's up to us to notice them.

March 15

Honoring His Father

"Those who honor their father will have joy in their children, and when they pray they are heard."

— Ben Sira (Sirach) 3:5

One of our dearest friends decided to give up his own home to live with his aging step-father. The whole family packed up and moved in with Dad. He's a little grouchy, set in his ways, and fusses about the new clutter. But my friend knows that the young grandchildren will be a source of life and laughter. And there will be more love than there ever was when his dad was alone.

MARCH 16

Fellowship of the Weak

"Compassion, to be with others when and where they suffer and to willingly enter into a fellowship of the weak, is God's way to justice and peace among people."

— Henri Nouwen, *Here and Now*

So often we try to win approval by proving we are powerful, or successful, or strong. Instead of trying to prove that we are worthy of love, Henri Nouwen suggests that we form a fellowship of the weak. We are *already* worthy of love, not because we have *proved* ourselves worthy, but simply because we are first loved by God. He created us out of love, so that we might also love one another.

March 17

Christ with Me

Feast of Saint Patrick

"I came to the Irish peoples to preach the Gospel and endure the taunts of unbelievers, putting up with reproaches . . . suffering many persecutions, even bondage, and losing my birthright of freedom for the benefit of others."

— Saint Patrick, *Confessions*

Saint Patrick, born into a British Christian family, was captured by Irish raiders and sold into slavery in Ireland. Yet he counted his trials as a gift, saying that while tending the flocks of his captors he used to pray constantly, and that the "love of God and the fear of him increased more and more and faith grew and the spirit was moved." He eventually escaped, but after studying for the priesthood, he had a vision in which he heard the Irish pleading with him, "Come and from now on walk with us." He returned to the country where he had been persecuted in order to evangelize and establish the faith.

Patrick teaches us to glorify God and give thanks, regardless of the circumstances. On his feast day, we can try to imitate this great saint. We can give thanks even when times are bad, when we feel persecuted, a slave to our jobs.

March 18

Wordless Angels

"See that you do not despise one of these little ones, for I say to you that their angels in heaven always look upon the face of my heavenly Father."

— Matthew 18:10

I am babysitting for my four-month-old grandson. Like my mom, he cannot speak. I spend the day gazing into his pure eyes, playing peek-a-boo, kissing his curly toes. How I love these wordless angels! Borrowing a phrase from Saint Augustine, we should bow down before them, because they are holy temples of the living God.

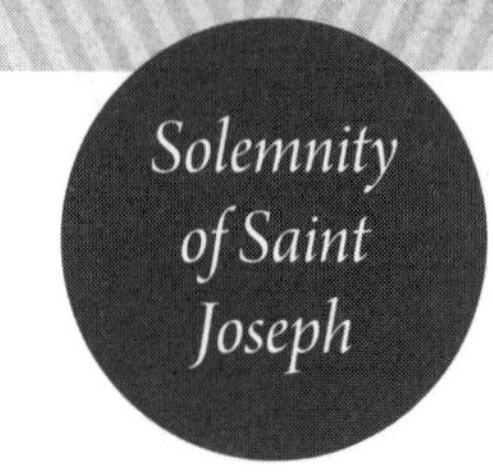

MARCH 19

Powerfully Unassuming

"Jacob the father of Joseph, the husband of Mary. Of her was born Jesus who is called the Messiah."

— Matthew 1:16

Notice how Joseph is sandwiched in between the great Old Testament figure and Mary, the mother of God, in Matthew's genealogy of Jesus. Quiet and unassuming Saint Joseph, whose words are not recorded in Scripture. But he serves and protects his family with humility, always trusting in God. And for this, he is truly great.

March 20

Standing By

"They divided his garments by casting lots. The people stood by and watched."

— Luke 23:34-35

It is hard to imagine that the people of Jerusalem were so immune to the brutality of crucifixion that they watched it as though it were an afternoon entertainment. The Son of God, the one who came to save us, is treated so vilely. Yet Jesus, in the form of the elderly, the handicapped, and the unborn, is discarded today, while so many of us stand by and watch.

March 21

Our Real Self

"Now one of the criminals hanging there reviled Jesus, saying, 'Are you not the Messiah? Save yourself and us.'"

— Luke 23:39

Perhaps it is part of our fallen human nature that we sometimes get angry with God. We forget how sinful we are and, like the criminal on the cross, demand that God fix everything *right now.* We can ask His forgiveness, though, when we have these lapses. And God probably prefers that we bring our real selves to Him in prayer. God doesn't want us making up pious platitudes.

March 22

Trusting God When It Makes No Sense

"He may throw me among strangers. He may make me feel desolate, make my spirits sink, hide my future from me — still He knows what He is about."

— Blessed John Henry Newman

The sharply dressed young man (he looks like he just stepped away from a high-level board meeting) is pacing, speaking *sotto voce* into his cell phone. "There's a woman in there who doesn't know who she is, crying out . . . " This must be his first time in a nursing home. "If I ever get to that point, just shoot me in the back of my head," he whispers angrily. I've had the same thought. What is the point of all this suffering, confusion, hanging on . . . especially if you don't even have sufficient faculties to offer up the suffering? But, as Cardinal Newman wrote, God knows what He is about. We have to trust.

March 23

Peace in the Midst of Despair

"No storm can shake my inmost calm,

While to that rock I'm clinging.

Since love is lord of heaven and earth

How can I keep from singing?"

— *My Life Flows On*, hymn

The elderly couple walks every day around the facility, rain or shine. He is pushing the wheelchair, she huddled under mountains of blankets when it's cold. I tell them that they are like the postal service: "Neither snow nor rain nor heat nor gloom of night stays these couriers from the swift completion of their appointed rounds." They are headed out back to their designated spot at the picnic table, where they play a daily game of backgammon. Every day I ask, "Who's winning?" And every day the answer is the same: "She's killing me." Their faithfulness throughout the storms of life, throughout illness and despair, inspires me. He is still strong enough to walk, and she is the backgammon queen.

March 24

When We Fall

"My most gentle Jesus,

how many times you have forgiven me;

and how many times I have fallen again and begun again to offend you!

By the merits of this second fall,

give me the grace to persevere in your love until death."

— Saint Alphonsus Liguori, *Stations of the Cross*

Tradition has it that Jesus fell three times while carrying the Cross to Calvary. Isaiah the prophet says that it was our infirmities that He bore, and our sufferings that He endured (see Is 53:4). Jesus fell, bearing the weight of our sins. We fall, too, even daily! The devil wants us to be sunk in despair over our failings, while Jesus says, "Let me take them."

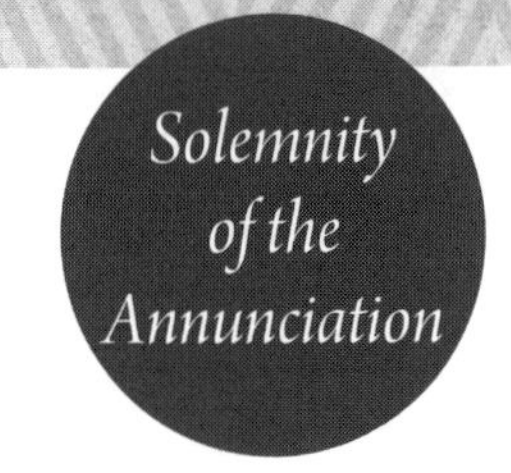

MARCH 25

Breath of God

"'The holy Spirit will come upon you, and the power of the Most High will overshadow you. Therefore the child to be born will be called holy, the Son of God.'"

— Luke 1:35

A hush settles over the dusty town of Nazareth and a late afternoon breeze, carrying the delicate scent of jasmine, stirs the young girl's cotton dress. All is quiet when the almighty God enters human history, when the gracious Word becomes flesh. No fanfare, no reporters, no royal-baby watch. Only stillness and openness to the breath of God. How much of God's action is hidden — unless we open our hearts to the possibility, as Mary did.

March 26

Interior Garden

"But when you pray, go to your inner room, close the door, and pray to your Father in secret."

— Matthew 6:6

What is our inner room like? Is it a quiet and peaceful room where we can hear the whisper of the Holy Spirit? Or is it noisy and demanding, filled with the clamor of the world? We should grow our inner room like a garden. Water it with grace from the sacraments, plant it with seeds from Scripture, fill it with the sunshine of compassion. And we can bring our inner garden with us wherever we go, to help brighten the days of those we meet.

MARCH 27

Suffering With

"To suffer with the other and for others . . . to suffer out of love and in order to become a person who truly loves . . . are we capable of this?"

— Pope Benedict XVI, *Spe Salvi*

Simon of Cyrene was dragged into the Passion. He didn't want to help Christ carry the Cross, but there he was. In the scene from the movie *The Passion of the Christ*, we see their arms entwined, Simon's and Jesus'. Simon gradually began to trust and became a true friend to Jesus along the way. Sometimes, caregivers are commissioned unwillingly, too. Yet, along the way, we discover Christ's love and mercy. We discover, too, that we are helping Christ, when we care for our loved ones in their time of suffering.

March 28

One Step at a Time

"The secret of waiting is the faith that the seed has been planted, that something has begun."

— Henri Nouwen, *Mornings with Henri Nouwen*

Irene's son is in the doghouse. His mom has applied for a job in New Hampshire, and he is discouraging her. He reminds his mom that she can't drive and she won't be able to take public transportation to get there. What a spoil sport! If they actually offer a job to the eighty-year-old stroke patient from the nursing home in Virginia, then we'll cross that bridge when we come to it. A woman needs her dreams.

March 29

Invitation to the Cross

"Rather, when you hold a banquet, invite the poor, the crippled, the lame, the blind; blessed indeed will you be because of their inability to repay you."

— Luke 14:13-14

Before Jesus' agony in the garden, Peter assured Him, "Lord, I am prepared to go to prison and to die with you" (Lk 22:33). Yet, a few hours later, Peter denied Him three times: I tell you, I do not even know the man!

How often are we exactly like Peter? We claim we love God, yet we turn away from the homeless man begging on the street. We are repulsed by the mindless and decrepit in the nursing homes. We are disgusted by the transgendered, offended by the incarcerated. We should pray that we have the strength to follow Jesus all the way to the Cross.

March 30

You've Got a Friend

"But God, who encourages the downcast, encouraged us by the arrival of Titus."

— 2 Corinthians 7:6

In the song *You've Got a Friend*, James Taylor sings that whenever we're down and troubled, even on the darkest night, we can call out and "I'll come running." Saint Paul was in exactly the same situation, and he wrote about it to the Corinthians. When he arrived in Macedonia, he was exhausted and under all kinds of stress — fears from within and quarrels with others. God sends us friends when we are reaching the limit of our strength. And on those days when you don't see even the sign of a friend, know that you can call on Jesus. He will come running.

March 31

Work

"Work, which Christ took up as something both redeemed and redeeming, becomes a means, a way of holiness, a specific task which sanctifies and can be sanctified."

— Saint Josemaria Escriva, *The Forge*

On Good Friday we venerate the Cross, singing "Behold the wood of the Cross, on which is hung our salvation." It is no coincidence that Jesus was a carpenter, daily working with wood, the material that becomes the instrument of His death. Perhaps we can meditate on our own work, on how through our daily tasks and humble duties we, too, can work out our own salvation when we unite them to Jesus.

April 1

Waiting out the Darkness

"He descended into hell. On the third day he rose again."

— Apostles' Creed

Jesus lay buried in the tomb for three days, and then the stone was rolled away. Those in nursing homes, those who are shut in or confined to bed, are like Jesus in the sepulcher. One day, the stone will be rolled away. We pray that God may give them — and us — the strength needed to wait for it.

April 2

God Is Dead?

"And behold, there was a great earthquake; for an angel of the Lord descended from heaven, approached, rolled back the stone, and sat upon it."

— Matthew 28:2

On Holy Saturday, we rent a garden tiller and turn over the dirt for our vegetable garden. The earth is dark and heavy, reminding us of the silence and stillness of the whole universe on the day Jesus went into the ground. For three days, God is dead. For some people, He remains dead, and they struggle with emptiness and meaninglessness, confusion and darkness. Until He is resurrected in their hearts again.

April 3

Brought to You by God

"For see, the winter is past,

the rains are over and gone.

The flowers appear on the earth,

the time of pruning the vines has come,

and the song of the dove is heard in our land."

— Song of Songs 2:11-12

On the first warm day of spring, we head outside, my mom in her wheelchair. Tulips in riotous colors greet us as soon as we exit the building. My mom spots a splash of yellow daffodils in the forest. Next, cherry blossoms! Then, we hear a cardinal sing. We are amazed at the wonder all around us, gifts from God that we might not otherwise have noticed. For someone in a wheelchair, who has no other form of entertainment, it's like visiting the Louvre or the pyramids of Egypt. We thank God for His gift of nature.

APRIL 4

The Sound of Silence

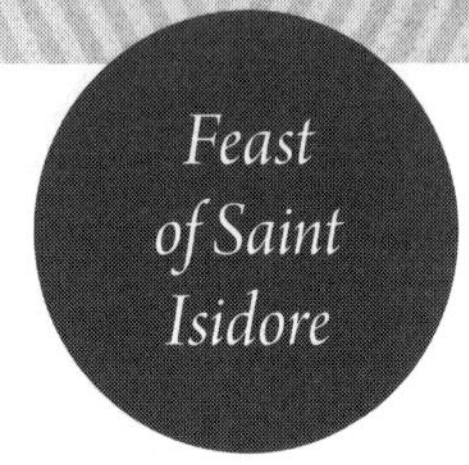

"When we pray, we talk to God; when we read [the Scriptures], God talks to us."

— Saint Isidore, *Book of Maxims*

I ask my mom to pray for my youngest daughter, who is hoping to go to Rome during the next school year. My mom expresses appropriate interest and concern over the prospect, though I am not quite sure how much she understands. Nonetheless, I believe her prayers are most powerful, especially because they are *not* verbal. In fact, her daily living is a prayer of suffering.

April 5

Good Samaritan

"But a Samaritan traveler who came upon him was moved with compassion at the sight. He approached the victim, poured oil and wine over his wounds and bandaged them. Then he lifted him up on his own animal, took him to an inn and cared for him."

— Luke 10:33-34

When the expert in the law wanted to justify himself, he asks Jesus, "And who is my neighbor?" He loves the *law*, not his actual neighbor. Jesus answers by showing him how to *be* a neighbor. You, too, are the Good Samaritan who tenderly cares for the suffering one, the one who cannot repay you.

April 6

Sage Advice

"You will surely wear yourself out, both you and these people with you. The task is too heavy for you; you cannot do it alone."

— Exodus 18:18

Everyone is depending on Moses to do everything, and it's taking its toll. His father-in-law tells him: this is not good, either for you or for those for whom you are responsible. Sometimes, you need help from other people. Sometimes, you need to delegate authority. I have nurses caring for my mom twenty-four hours of the day. I truly wish I could do it myself, but right now I need help. My cousins on the other side of the country help me care for my mom's house so that I can be with her daily. It's good to accept help when we need it.

April 7

Usefulness

"He saved us and called us to a holy life, not according to our works but according to his own design."

— 2 Timothy 1:9

Our preoccupation with technology (faster, better, more apps!) certainly affects our understanding of the world. How often do we think solely in mechanistic terms, functions and processes, instrumentality? The real danger is losing our sense of our true purpose and true dignity. We risk valuing only what this or that person can *do*. The folks in the nursing home can't do much. Nonetheless, they have a very serious and significant purpose. But, we have to see beyond functionality and utility.

April 8

Good Works

"What good is it, my brothers, if someone says he has faith but does not have works?"

— James 2:14

Often, we pray so that we might do good works, or that our work will be blessed. But one spiritual writer suggests that the opposite is even better. Do good works *so that* your prayer will be improved! I resolve to give this a try.

April 9

Uprooting Bitterness

"He has made my teeth grind on gravel,

and made me cower in ashes;

my soul is bereft of peace,

I have forgotten what happiness is."

— Lamentations 3:16-17, RSVCE

Mrs. X. has lost all her front teeth, and she tells me that this is ironic since her late husband was a dentist. She inches her wheelchair forward, using her slippered feet. "Nobody does anything for me," she complains. I offer to push her wheelchair, and she refuses. "I need some exercise, because I never leave this place." Let us pray today for God's peace to enter the hearts of all the lonely and bitter ones, the ones who have forgotten what happiness is.

April 10

The Boulder

"Taking the body, Joseph wrapped it [in] clean linen and laid it in his new tomb that he had hewn in the rock. Then he rolled a huge stone across the entrance to the tomb and departed. But Mary Magdalene and the other Mary remained sitting there, facing the tomb."

— Matthew 27:59-61

You can just imagine the scene: two women, dumb in their grief and despair, staring glumly at the boulder in front of them. All they can see is that barricade. How often do our problems and responsibilities weigh on us like a giant stone and see no possibility of changing things? Yet, any moment, any hour now, an angel will come to roll away the rock. Let's try to remember this: don't look at the boulder of despair. Trust that Jesus will soon appear.

April 11

Clouds and Hope

"Cloud-puffball, torn tufts, tossed pillows flaunt forth."

— Gerard Manley Hopkins, *That Nature is a Heraclitean Fire and of the Comfort of the Resurrection*

Yesterday was cold, dreary, sleeting. Everything was dismal, heavy. The end of the world is surely coming. Desolation! Flee to the mountains! Of course, today dawns bright and sunny, the clouds scampering happily across periwinkle sky. Hope rises in my heart, like the puffball clouds. God writes His story of salvation on all creation. After the Cross, comes the Resurrection.

April 12

A Mission

"May the favor of the Lord our God be ours.

Prosper the work of our hands!

Prosper the work of our hands!"

— Psalm 90:17

The old man skillfully maneuvers his wheelchair between all the other residents' wheelchairs, propelling himself with his feet, like Fred Flintstone driving his car. "Should I move out of your way?" I ask. No, he tells me. He can do it! He goes two feet, reaches the wastebasket, and tosses his napkin in with flair. He returns breathless, feet pumping. "Mission accomplished!" he announces with wry humor. Each of us has a mission in life, a purpose that God has ordained. Each day it unfolds as we pray for God's blessing on our work.

April 13

Angels in the Tomb

"But Mary stayed outside the tomb weeping. And as she wept, she bent over into the tomb and saw two angels in white sitting there."

— John 20:11-12

In the midst of her sorrow, as she is weeping, Mary Magdalene peers into the tomb and sees the angels. Yet still, she is not consoled. How often does this happen to us? When we are in the midst of suffering, when we are grieving or even despairing, we see nothing but an empty tomb. The empty tomb of dashed hopes, the empty tomb of a bad relationship, the empty tomb of a sick loved one. Yet, with eyes of faith, the tomb isn't empty after all. There are angels sitting there!

April 14

Pruning

"He takes away every branch in me that does not bear fruit, and everyone that does he prunes so that it bears more fruit."

— John 15:2

My daughter starts whacking away at the wyeberry bush with the pruning shears. As the pile of branches grows higher at her feet, I worry that we will have no berries this year. "Don't worry, Mom," she says. "See these branches? They are all dead! The berries will grow from the new shoots that were sent out last year. We'll have even more berries than last year!" With illness and with caregiving, God is pruning our branches.

April 15

All for You

"This is my commandment: love one another as I love you."

— John 15:12

Pause for a moment to think about the fact that Jesus suffered and died on the Cross for you. Not you plural, but you singular. Every drop of blood He shed, He shed for you. He would have done so even if you were the only living person. When we really take this to heart, we realize that every moment we care for another person, we are doing exactly what Jesus did, and what He wants us to do.

April 16

Ocean of Mercy

"I pour out a whole ocean of graces upon those souls who approach the fount of my mercy."

— Saint Faustina, *Diary*

Saint Faustina teaches us to say, "Jesus, I trust in you." We need to repeat these words so that they sink deep into our hearts. We say we trust God, but we stay up nights worrying. We say we trust, but we rush to check items off our to-do list. We could have spent an hour in the adoration chapel. When we really trust, we will find peace.

April 17

Living only in the Father

"Amma Syncletica said, " . . . 'We are like exiles: we have been separated from the things of this world and have given ourselves in one faith to the one Father. We need nothing of what we have left behind.'"

— *Daily Readings with the Desert Fathers*

I return to my parents' beloved home beneath the rugged Sierra Nevada's and the expansive clear sky. I divide up their belongings into those I will bring back with me and those I must sell or give away. It's a wretched business, and my only consolation is that my mom does not know. Our Lord, with His divine understanding, knew everything that would happen to Him. And this must have caused even greater pain and suffering. Yet, He placed himself entirely in the hands of His Father. When you're feeling as though you are an exile (day after day in the sickroom) or your memories are too painful, place yourself with Jesus in the Garden of Gethsemane, in the hands of the Father.

April 18

Who's Blessing Whom?

"How is it possible to keep nursing the sick when they are not getting better? How can I keep consoling the dying when their deaths only bring me more grief? The answer is that they all hold a blessing for me, a blessing that I need to receive."

— Henri Nouwen, *The Spiritual Life*

We are caring for the sick — yes, of course. But mysteriously, they also are caring for us.

April 19

Father God

"They did not know that I cared for them. . . .
I fostered them like those
who raise an infant to their cheeks;
I bent down to feed them."

— Hosea 11:3-4

We see the tenderness of God in these lines. When I pick up my grandchild and kiss his soft cheek and gently rock him to sleep, I cannot imagine loving anyone more. And this is how God feels about us! Yet, so often we think of God in punitive terms, as though He is an ogre who lays in wait for us to make a false step. We assume He wants to pounce on us and punish us. Rather, He wants to hold us and heal us.

April 20

Cotton-Candy Canopy

"The sweetness of the hidden God is the delight of life."

— Frederick William Faber, *Spiritual Conferences*

When the wind blows the cherry blossoms, they swirl through the air like pink snow. A cherry tree in peak bloom looks like a cloud of cotton candy atop a tree trunk, a fountain of pink sweetness. My mom exclaims at the pink surprise. Each day, a new tree is in full bloom. I park the wheelchair directly under the laden branches of delight for a glimpse of heaven, a glimpse of God's beauty.

April 21

God Awaits

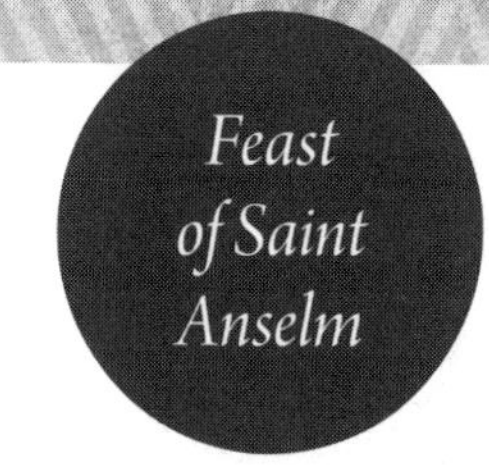

"Cast aside, now, your burdensome cares, and put away your toilsome business. Yield room for some little time to God; and rest for a little time in him."

— Saint Anselm, *The Prosologian*

Saint Anselm's motto was "faith seeking understanding." What the great philosopher and theologian meant was that his work, borne out of his love for God, sought a deeper understanding of his beloved. This brilliant man was also very tender. It is said that once a frightened rabbit being pursued by dogs hid beneath his horse's hooves. While everyone laughed, Anselm wept.

O Jesus, meek and humble of heart, make my heart like yours!

April 22

Walking Partner

"And it happened that while they were conversing and debating, Jesus himself drew near and walked with them."

— Luke 24:15

The disciples were discouraged, because all their hopes are dashed. They had expected that Jesus would be the one to redeem Israel. They didn't realize they had something better: the risen Lord himself walking with them. How often do we focus so intently on having things go our way that we fail to see the better thing happening right now?

April 23

Enlarging the Heart

"Make me feel as thou hast felt;

Make my soul to glow and melt

With the love of Christ our Lord."

— *Stabat Mater*

I read a news article about a tiny baby who lived less than a year with a fatal condition called spinal muscular atrophy. Throughout his short life, he required round-the-clock care. His parents never regretted the great sacrifices they had to make to care for him. He also gave love. Hundreds attended the funeral, confessions were heard, and relatives came back to the faith. Why does God allow the innocent to suffer? This mystery is answered only by the hearts that are now grown larger, more compassionate, and more filled with Christ's love.

April 24

Hidden Jesus

"Jesus said to her, 'Woman, why are you weeping? Whom are you looking for?' She thought it was the gardener."

— John 20:15

How often when we are feeling sad, exhausted, stressed out, or burdened, do we fail to see Jesus in front of us? He appears so subtly. He is the sick person we are caring for (there He is!), the illegal immigrant who mows the grounds, the simple Communion bread.

Feast of Saint Mark

April 25

Urgent Call

"He will raise a signal to a far-off nation,

and whistle for it from the ends of the earth.

Then speedily and promptly they will come."

— Isaiah 5:26

Saint Mark skips right past a lengthy genealogy and the story of Jesus' birth to get straight to the point. In the very first chapter of his Gospel he writes, "And the Spirit immediately drove him out into the wilderness" (v. 13); "immediately they left their nets" (v. 18); "immediately he called them" (v.20) and "they went into Capernaum; and immediately on the Sabbath" (v. 21) (RSVCE). Things happen quickly under the power of the Holy Spirit, and Mark captures that force, that immediacy, that urgency. Are we as quick to answer God when He calls us?

April 26

Hands of Jesus

"Ascension is the gesture of blessing. The hands of Christ have become the ceiling that covers us and at the same time have become the effective power that opens the door of the world toward what is above."

— Cardinal Joseph Ratzinger, *Images of Hope*

We are likely puzzled by the joy the disciples feel upon Christ's Ascension. Christ is leaving them (again) but this time it's different. Pope Benedict tells us that His final gesture is one of blessing. In the blessing, He leaves, but in the blessing, He also remains.

Father places both his large hands on my mom's forehead, and says, " Don't be afraid." This blessing, truly effective, remains with her. It opens the door of heaven and calls down God's own peace and healing.

April 27

Bearing Fruit for All

"The term 'communion of saints' refers also to the communion of 'holy persons' (sancti) *in Christ who 'died for all,' so that what each one does or suffers in and for Christ bears fruit for all."*

— *Catechism of the Catholic Church*, 961

One day Father Pierre Favre, one of the first Jesuits, was struck by the sight of poor beggars covered with sores. Even if he didn't have money to give them, couldn't he have begged for some? At that moment, he prayed to the "spirits of all the wretched in this world" who had died. He prayed that they would advocate for the poor and would pray for *him*, that he would have the grace to care for *them*.

What a beautiful thought! When we feel discouraged by the fact that we haven't done enough for those who need our care, we can pray to all the sick and poor who are now in heaven. We can also pray to the guardian angels of those for whom we care.

April 28

You Can Do It!

"When ridiculed, we bless; when persecuted, we endure; when slandered, we respond gently."

— 1 Corinthians 4:12-13

How do you respond when someone criticizes you, disagrees with you, shuns you, or slanders you? Do you get angry, irritated, or retaliate? It's a normal human response! Yet, spiritual writers tell us that these are occasions to grow in holiness. Not only can you refuse to succumb to irritation, but you can *embrace* those occasions. They become opportunities to be like Christ when He prayed as He hung from the cross, "Father, forgive them, they know not what they do."

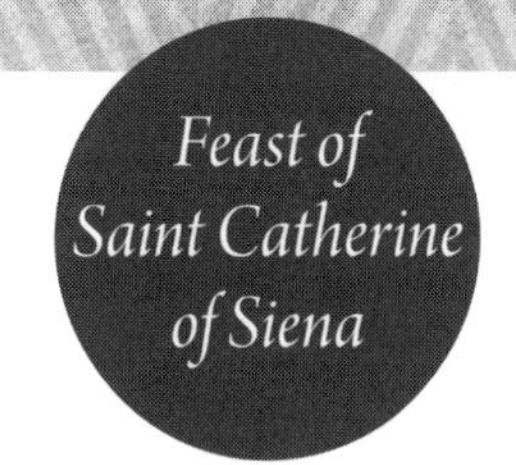

April 29

Two Crowns

"'There cannot be love of Me, without love of the neighbor, nor love of the neighbor without love of Me.'"

— Saint Catherine, *Dialogue*

In a vision, Jesus offered Catherine two crowns. One was a crown of gold, and the other was a crown of thorns. Catherine chose the crown of thorns. It meant she chose the more difficult, more humble, yet more loving path. That turned out to include visiting prisoners condemned to death, accompanying them to their executions, burying the victims of plague, nursing the sick, and taking on the cases nobody else wanted.

Saint Catherine, pray for us, so that we will have the strength to choose the more difficult path.

April 30

Covering the Bases

"Let your love for one another be intense, because love covers a multitude of sins."

— 1 Peter 4:8

Another translation of this Scripture passage reads: "Let your love be constant." I am striving for both: constant and intense love. Because, Lord knows, I have a multitude of sins.

May 1

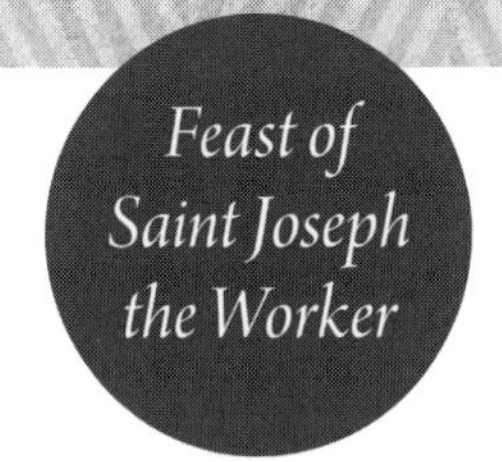

Secret Joy

"[Saint Joseph] too knew the humble, secret joy of duty done, and of all the trials and hardships of daily toil endured."

— Saint John XXIII, *Prayers and Devotions*

Even in the Garden of Eden, the first man and woman worked. God gave Adam and Eve the garden, and asked them to cultivate and care for it. Today, we honor Saint Joseph the Worker. He cared for the Holy Family and worked hard to provide for them. There is little written in Scripture about Saint Joseph, except that he was a carpenter and a just man, a man of faith. God honors those who work humbly, silently, and faithfully — even if unrecognized by the world.

MAY 2

Mary and the Eucharist

"When we say that in the Eucharist we have the Son and in Mary we have his Mother, have we not said it all?"

— Saint John XXIII, *Prayers and Devotions*

There is a beautiful painting, *The Virgin Adoring the Host*, by Jean-Auguste-Dominique Ingres. Mary contemplates the sacred host atop a chalice. Her hands are folded in prayer, the tranquility of her lovely face a mirror of the Eucharist. The first time I saw this painting, I was startled. I had never thought of Mary receiving Communion. Just as she received her Son as a divine spark of life at the Annunciation, so, too, she would have received him in her later years, in Holy Communion. We can be grateful today for Mary, Mother of the Church, and our mother, too. We also thank God for her Son, whom we can receive, just as she did, in Holy Communion.

May 3

Forgetting

"Remember that my life is like the wind."

— Job 7:7

The elderly gentleman, elegantly attired and carrying a cane, leaned against the reception desk at the assisted living facility where he lives. "Tell me, darlin'," he said in a dignified Southern drawl, "Is the bridge game today?"

"Yes, Mr. Lacy, at 2 p.m."

"Thank you, darlin', and might I ask, where the bridge game is held?"

"It's just upstairs, in the lounge on the second floor."

"Ah," he replied as he adjusted his cufflinks. "And where would that be, again?"

When I overheard this, I thought of Saint Ignatius. In a well-known prayer, he offered God everything: his will, his liberty, his memory. "Give me only your love and your grace. That is enough for me."

This is a scary way to pray. We don't want to lose our memories and our liberty. But really, we are scared because we don't truly believe in the immensity of God's love. Let's pray that we can accept God's love and grace.

May 4

Be the One

"Be the one ... be the one who will satiate the Thirst. Instead of saying 'I thirst' say 'be the one.'"

— Mother Teresa, *Come Be My Light*

Blessed Teresa of Calcutta prayed that she might be able to console Jesus during his agony on the Cross, specifically in his thirst for souls. She wanted to go into the "dark holes" of the streets of Calcutta, where the poor and diseased lay abandoned. She watned to bring the light of Christ to them. As a caregiver, you follow Mother Teresa in doing small things with great love. You, too, console Jesus in His thirst for love.

MAY 5

Gardening

"What is all this juice and all this joy?

A strain of the earth's sweet being in the beginning

In Eden garden . . ."

— Gerard Manley Hopkins, *Spring*

Gardens are significant. Paradise was a garden, where God would walk in the breezy time of day. When our hearts lift at the sight of the first bud, is that perhaps a hearkening back to original bliss in the Garden of Eden? Now, that garden remains hidden behind the wings of the Cherubim and the flaming sword. So, we have to go about the humble work of gardening. We must work the soil, plant our seeds, and wait. Seeds of faith, of suffering, of our mortal bodies are planted in the darkness. One day, these seeds will spring forth, bursting into the sunlight, all transformed. Transformed into joy, into new life. Let's embrace the gardening.

May 6

Eternity Dwelling in Us

"The picture of Mary's later life serves us as promise and security. It shows us that we must not take time too seriously, for if we have faith, eternity dwells in us."

— Romano Guardini, *The Rosary of Our Lady*

There were many years, perhaps, following the crucifixion, death, and resurrection of Our Lord, when Mary remained on this earth. Father Guardini writes that Mary was waiting for her Son to call her home. But, her waiting was in complete tranquility, total fulfillment. I pray that the time of waiting my mom endures is filled with similar tranquility and a sense of indwelling eternity. And for all those who wait — the sick, the elderly, the shut-ins, the imprisoned — let's ask the Blessed Mother to give them a sense of her peace.

May 7

God-Particles

"We are in the month of May: what could be found more beautiful and more encouraging than a visit to the altar of Mary, there to join our voices with the songs of spring."

— Saint John XXIII, *Prayers and Devotions*

It's a minor miracle when I can take my mom outside for a wheelchair stroll. When she feels well enough to endure the Hoyer Lift, there are two nursing assistants available to do the lifting. But this happens only when the weather is gentle. I relish these opportunities even more than I used to enjoy the big occasions — the anniversary celebrations or the family gatherings. I see things now in small moments of grace. These are atoms of grace, God-particles of grace!

On a day like today, everything is serendipitous. Birds are chirping as we catch sight of a busy squirrel. My mom waves to the gardener like he's an old friend. We marvel at the height of the trees and the warmth of the sun on our faces. Every day, we can experience these small miracles, these tokens of God's presence, if only we would pay attention.

May 8

Casting the Net

"If God were to say to you right now, 'Throw your net on the starboard side of the boat,' would you cling to it saying, 'Oh Lord, the timing is not right'? Or would you say, 'Lord, I just couldn't do that, people will think I'm nuts'? You have to be willing, in your interior life, to throw your net on the starboard side every day of your life."

— *Mother Angelica's Private and Pithy Lessons from the Scriptures*

The disciples have been up all night fishing. They are hungry, wet, and cold. And they have no fish. The mysterious man on the shore gently teases them — "Children, have you caught no fish?" He tells them to cast their nets once more, on the starboard side. (This is so they will know their success is due to Jesus' help, not their fishing prowess!) They bring in their biggest catch ever. But here is the best part. Waiting on the shore is Jesus, grill master, cooking the hungry men breakfast. He is serving crispy charcoal-broiled fish, crusty warm bread. What delicate charity, such loving attention to detail! He cares for us just like this, every day.

May 9

An Ever-Present Help

"Bruis'd, derided, curs'd, defil'd,

She beheld her tender child

All with bloody scourges rent."

— *Stabat Mater*

It is so painful to stand by while a loved one suffers a debilitating disease, a terminal illness, or a lifelong disability. But, this puts us in good company, with the Blessed Mother as she followed her son's way of the cross. Mary did not become bitter or hardened as a result. She remained faithful, by her son throughout. Let us pray to Our Lady that we become like her: gentle, patient, persevering.

May 10

Feast of Saint Damien of Molokai

Consoling the Lepers

"Here I am in the midst of my dear lepers. They are so frightful to see, it is true, but they have souls redeemed at the price of the precious blood of our Divine Savior. He also in his divine charity consoled lepers. If I cannot cure them as he did, at least I can console them."

— Saint Damien de Veuster, *Letters*

Like Christ, Damien de Veuster lived among those he wished to heal. Then, like Jesus, Damien became an outcast. He contracted leprosy. Despite being completely cut off from all society, isolated on the island of Molokai, he writes that serving these poor souls was his "greatest happiness." We can ask Saint Damien to pray for us, that we might have such a generous heart with which to console the sick.

May 11

Downward Mobility!

"The compassionate life is the life of downward mobility!"

— Henri Nouwen, *Here and Now*

Why would anyone want to hang around the poor, the diseased, the outcasts of society, the homeless, the fringe groups? Yet, Jorge Mario Bergoglio, now Pope Francis, spent his eighteen years as bishop and cardinal in Buenos Aires doing just that. A priest from the slums said that Father Bergoglio would just show up, wander around the alleys, and talk with people. It's estimated that over the years he personally spoke with over half the people in those areas. An aide said that the future pope saw the poor and needy not as people he could help, but rather "as people from whom he could learn."

The compassionate life — the life of the caregiver — is the life of listening and learning.

May 12

Praising God

"A monk's cell is like the furnace of Babylon where the three children found the Son of God, and it is like the pillar of cloud where God spoke with Moses."

— *Daily Readings with the Desert Fathers*

I read to my mom, even though she looks as though she'd rather nap. I choose one of her favorite Old Testament stories: King Nebuchadnezzar and the fiery furnace. The repetition of the melodious names — Shadrach, Meshach and Abednego — and the powerful rhythm of the passage mesmerize her. "If our God . . . can save us from the white-hot furnace and from your hands, O king, may he save us! But even if he will not, you should know, O king, that we will not serve your god!" (Dn 3:17-18).

We can pray this way, too. Save us, Lord! But even if You choose not to save us from this earthly pain, we praise You.

May 13

Feast of Our Lady of Fátima

Bring Souls to Christ and Christ to Souls

"Do whatever he tells you."

— John 2:5

Some folks like to speculate about the mysterious third secret of Fátima. They wonder if it has been fully revealed and whether or not Mary's heavenly requests have been fulfilled. Such speculation sidetracks us. In any case, we can continue to do as Mary always does: bring souls to Christ. We can do this through our prayers, and we can do this through our work. Even the smallest task you perform, if you do it with love, helps grow Christ's love in the world.

May 14

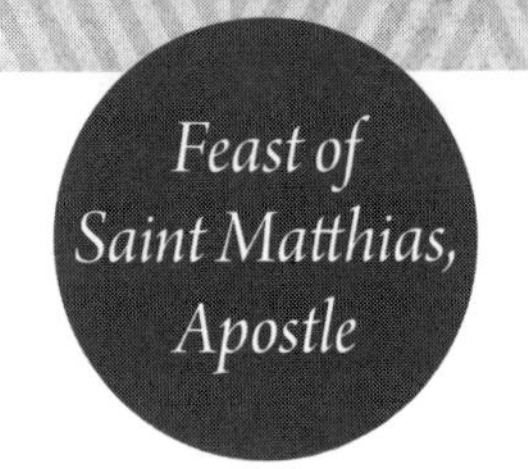

Send Me!

"Then I heard the voice of the Lord saying, 'Whom shall I send? Who will go for us?' 'Here I am,' I said; 'send me!'"

— Isaiah 6:8

Saint Matthias had been a witness to the Resurrected Christ. So, he was chosen to take the place of the traitor Judas (see Acts 1:15-26). Perhaps there are supernatural substitutions of good over evil everywhere. Most, perhaps, are hidden and unheralded. There are opportunities, accessible to each of us. We can substitute the healing balm of God's love, for example, for the wounds left by another's rudeness or spitefulness. Maybe we are chosen by God today to make just such a substitution. Perhaps we can replace unkindness and hatred with goodness and peace.

May 15

Feast of Saint Isidore the Farmer

Day-Laboring Angels

"He knows that he has nothing of himself, but that everything comes from God, and that he is unable to do anything without divine grace."

— Romano Guardini, *The Rosary of Our Lady*

Saint Isidore was a simple day laborer who worked on a wealthy Spaniard's farm. He would attend morning Mass daily, and this would make him late to work. Yet, he never neglected any of his duties. It is said that he would send his guardian angel ahead of him and sometimes there were two angels seen helping him plow the fields. He is a saint for those who wish to offer God their manual labor and their ordinary work. And, like Isidore, we can ask our guardian angels to help us in our daily tasks.

May 16

Pierced by a Sword

"(And you yourself a sword will pierce) so that the thoughts of many hearts may be revealed."

— Luke 2:35

On this beautiful day, when Joseph and Mary present their baby in the temple, Mary receives this startling and disturbing news. It is a prophecy that she will ponder for the next thirty years. If I had received such a word, it would have been like a dark cloud of doom hovering over my life. When ominous clouds of worry and bad news threaten to steal our joy, we can turn to Mary. She knew how to hold these things in her heart, never letting them disturb her peace.

May 17

Facebook Friends

"Our hope for you is firm, for we know that as you share in our sufferings, you also share in the encouragement."

— 2 Corinthians 1:7

My friend Mary will reach out to her Facebook friends when her daughter Courtney needs prayers. Then, the Facebook friends storm heaven. It is consoling to think that we might be helping in our friend's time of need. We see the power of the Body of Christ happening in real time on Facebook. Mary feels lifted up in prayer, and we are united as a community of compassion. Mary tells us that she can feel our prayers!

May 18

The Door of Humility

"For humility is the door to the kingdom, opening up to those who come near."

— John Climacus, *The Ladder of Divine Ascent*

My friend Chris says that things began to go downhill just as she turned eighty. One day, she fell, right outside of IHOP. Three young men came rushing to her rescue: a Marine, a paramedic, and "a hunk," she laughs ruefully. They helped her up and offered to call an ambulance. "No!" she exclaimed, "I have to meet my friends for breakfast!" Chris says it's all part of God's plan. These humiliations help her grow in the virtue of humility. And humility is the door to the Kingdom.

MAY 19

The Dark Cistern

"'Look, I had another dream,' he said; 'this time, the sun and the moon and eleven stars were bowing down to me.'"

— Genesis 37:9

Israel's son Joseph was so naïve! He told his dreams to his brothers, and they became envious and plotted to kill him. Fortunately, they decided to sell him into slavery instead. But, see how God turns evil into good. In the end, when famine came to the land, Joseph saved his brothers and his whole family from starvation. Yet, who could have guessed when Joseph was thrown into the dark cistern that the outcome would be so marvelous? Next time you find yourself in a dark cistern, like Joseph, remember that God always brings good out of evil.

May 20

Karma

"Each solitary kind action that is done, the whole world over, is working briskly in its own sphere to restore the balance between right and wrong."

— Frederick William Faber, *Spiritual Conferences*

I step in front of the tall Indian man, inadvertently taking the spot in the front of the line at Starbucks. I apologize immediately and wave him forward, but he demurs graciously. "No, please, you go first!" I thank him, and he says with a melodious voice and twinkling eyes, "It always comes back, you know!" Later, when his caramel macchiato is called, I fetch it and bring it to him. "See!" he cries delightedly, "What did I tell you?"

May 21

The Saving Calm

"By waiting and by calm you shall be saved,
in quiet and in trust shall be your strength."

— Isaiah 30:15

I enter the silent space. It's such a relief to be away from the busyness and noise of the world, the anxiety and stress that follow me everywhere, except here. I step into stillness, bow down before the Lord. The Lord is present here, disguised in the monstrance. But, this is how I know He is here. You will find no more perfect calm, no more peace, no more relaxation — not even at a spa or a hotel on the beach — than you find here. That is the proof.

May 22

Becoming Real

"Generally, by the time you are Real, most of your hair has been loved off, and your eyes drop out and you get all loose in the joints and very shabby. But these things don't matter at all, because once you are Real you can't be ugly, except to people who don't understand."

— Margery Williams, *The Velveteen Rabbit*

We are trying to battle middle-age spread by working out at a nearby gym several nights a week. I run on the treadmill, and he rides the stationery bike. All around us are young people looking at themselves in the mirror as they lift weights or take part in a Zumba workout, though they are already skinny and buff. All this attention to our appearance! Will we lose the ability to recognize the Real?

Feast of Saint Crispin of Viterbo

May 23

The Little Beast of Burden

"A brother asked one of the elders, saying: There are two brothers, of whom one remains praying in his cell, fasting six days at a time and doing a great deal of penance. The other one takes care of the sick. Which one's work is more pleasing to God? The elder replied: If that brother who fasts six days at a time were to hang himself up by the nose, he could not equal the one who takes care of the sick."

— Thomas Merton, *The Wisdom of the Desert*

There is a nurse who spends her days at her desk writing up reports and ordering underlings to care for the patients. She is like the Pharisees whom Jesus denounced when he said that they "tie up heavy burdens . . . lay them on people's shoulders" (Mt 23:4). Saint Crispin of Viterbo, a Franciscan lay brother, was just the opposite. He called himself "the little beast of burden of the Capuchins." He dug the garden, cooked for his brother monks, and cared for the sick. And he became a saint in the process.

MAY 24

Panic Solves Nothing

"But they did not understand what he said to them."

— Luke 2:50

Have you ever lost a small child while shopping? I remember when my oldest was just two years old, and how I panicked! Then I found her, laughing and hiding in the middle of a clothing rack. Can you imagine how Mary and Joseph felt when they lost Jesus? And when they found Him, He explained that He had to be in His Father's house. They didn't understand, yet they believed and trusted. And so it is with us, too. Those days when we are fearful and anxious, when we feel we might have lost Jesus, we just have to trust.

May 25

Feeling Forgotten

"'When will he die and his name be forgotten?'
When someone comes to visit me, he speaks
without sincerity. . . .
They imagine the worst about me:
'He has had ruin poured over him;
That one lying down will never rise again.'"

— Psalm 41:6-8

Mrs. X. is miserable because she thinks she has been left alone to die in the nursing home. The elderly and bedridden can feel as though they no longer have any purpose in life, that they are useless to themselves and to others, and that they might as well die. Yet, even the most infirm, those who cannot speak or do anything for themselves, are hugely significant in God's eyes. Jesus himself was once naked, scorned, and left for dead. He (yes, God!) suffered all this so that, mysteriously, we would not disdain or despair of any moment of our lives. No matter how crushingly humiliating and senseless it may seem. Each one of us is loved madly by God, considered by Him to be a priceless pearl.

May 26

Strength for the Journey

"This last anointing fortifies the end of our earthly life like a solid rampart for the final struggles before entering the Father's house."

— *Catechism of the Catholic Church*, 1523

At one hundred years old, Moses climbs Mount Nebo at God's bidding, to take in a spectacular view of the Promised Land. He sees below him the land of Gilead, the palms of Jericho, and all the way to the Western Sea. He feels the warmth of the sun, the cool breeze scented with sage and other desert grasses. And he bids all this farewell. In the wisdom of old age, Moses sees not only the physical beauty of the land, but also the reality of God's faithfulness.

The Sacrament of the Anointing of the Sick prepares us for our final journey in life. We are anointed at baptism as we begin our Christian journey, and we are anointed at the end. This sacrament gives us strength and courage to climb that last mountain.

May 27

The Greatest Fear

"If isolation means not being loved, being abandoned, being alone on one's own, this situation is indeed the fear underlying all our fears."

— Cardinal Joseph Ratzinger, *God and the World*

It's been two weeks of beautiful weather, and I haven't seen Dr. Lillian on her usual bench in the sun. She's my mom's age, but is capable of living on her own. But she has no family left, so she likes it here with the other elderly folk who need assistance. Finally, on Mother's Day, she's back in her usual spot. I wish her "Happy Mother's Day." She says, "Let's call it Easter," and then asks, "Does the judge who used to visit his mother every day for lunch ever wonder about that old woman who always sits on the bench?" I reassure her: "I wonder about you! I missed you when you were gone!" She smiles, but there's such sadness in her eyes.

May 28

New and Old Treasures

"For although you have hidden these things from the wise and the learned you have revealed them to the childlike."

— Luke 10:21

As I stroll with my grandchild along the old railroad trail, pointing out the tulips, cars, and bicyclists, I am struck by the fact that I do the same when I stroll with my mom in her wheelchair. The simplest things of life and nature bring such joy to both the new and the old. Jesus says the disciple of the Kingdom is like the homeowner who brings treasure both new and old out of his storeroom (see Mt 13:52). These treasures — both new and old — point us toward the kingdom of God.

May 29

Composted Sin

"Fire, like love, knows no bounds. . . . The fire that came upon their heads consumed their hard-heartedness, their weaknesses, their fear, and their lukewarmness. Pentecost is an influx of Someone Who is Love."

— *Mother Angelica's Private and Pithy Lessons from the Scriptures*

We have a compost bin that steams when it's really working well. All the vegetable scraps, the egg shells, the kitchen waste disappear and become rich, dark, earth. This is sort of like purgatory. In purgatory, our sins are steamed away. The scraps of our life that we thought were important, but really were just distractions, decay. The wasted time, the shells of indifference to God's love. All eventually becomes a rich, fruitful foundation, capable of new growth.

May 30

Come, Holy Spirit!

"Then there appeared to them tongues as of fire, which parted and came to rest on each one of them."

— Acts 2:3

The tongues of fire rested on each one. Each of us receives the Holy Spirit in our own unique way. Some may receive the gift of counseling, others the gift of piety, still others wisdom. But all come from the same God, so we are drawn together in unity. The activity ladies at the nursing home have the gift of friendliness, inspiration, and good cheer. With something new and interesting each day, they raise the spirits of the residents. Let's ask the Holy Spirit to stir into flame His gifts in us!

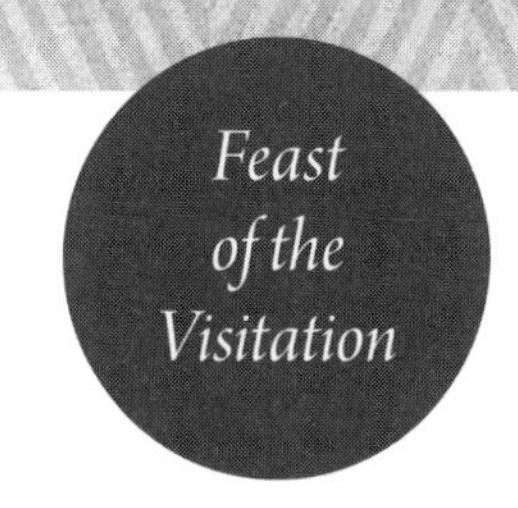

May 31

Cousinly Consolation

"My soul proclaims the greatness of the Lord;
my spirit rejoices in God my savior."

— Luke 1:46-47

When Mary hears that her older cousin Elizabeth is pregnant, she leaves *in haste* to visit her, to serve her. My cousins, too, are so generous with their time. They come nearly every day to visit their aunt, my mother. They bring stories, and photos, and hand-knit sweaters. They bring such light and warmth. I am sure the Blessed Mother was just like that, too.

June 1

Finding Shelter

"How many times I yearned to gather your children together, as a hen gathers her young under her wings."

— Matthew 23:37

Jesus *wept* over Jerusalem; He compared himself to a mother. Such was the tenderness of His heart. And yet, we doubt Him. We think He has abandoned us to a miserable fate. We wonder where He is going with all this suffering and these trials. We wait for the other shoe to drop. Instead, let Him gather us under the wings of His Sacred Heart.

JUNE 2

Being Led

"Amen, amen, I say to you, when you were younger, you used to dress yourself and go where you wanted; but when you grow old, you will stretch out your hands, and someone else will dress you and lead you where you do not want to go."

— John 21:18

The counselor asks me whether my mom indicated her preferences when it comes to getting dressed. My mom had always been quite elegantly dressed, and she had strong opinions about style. But now she allows the nursing assistants to choose her clothing for the day. It's sad to see how many aspects of her personality are disappearing. Is this yet one more earthly attachment to renounce? Does this somehow fit into her mission during these final years? At least we discover that she looks fantastic in crimson, a color she never used to wear.

June 3

Christ Within Me, Christ Before Me

"Yet I live, no longer I, but Christ lives in me."

— Galatians 2:20

In the slums of Calcutta, Mother Teresa did not see simply the masses of starving and dying who lay in the streets. She saw Christ through the eyes of Christ. And when she gently held a dying child or nursed a leper, they saw Christ in that person. Perhaps this is another example of God's omnipresence, His immensity.

June 4

In the Belly of the Beast

"For he afflicts and shows mercy,

casts down to the depths of Hades,

brings up from the great abyss."

— Tobit 13:2

Jonah was in the belly of the whale for three days, prefiguring Jesus in the darkness of the tomb. If you stay too long in the darkness deep in the earth, in the caverns that have no light within, you will go blind. When we are in such darkness, in the depths of the sea of sadness, in the belly of the monster, we can't see the way out, and we feel close to despair. But take heart. The whale spat Jonah up onto the shore. Jesus rose from the dead, and we will find joy again. There is light at the end of this tunnel.

JUNE 5

Carpe Diem

"Man's great, true hope which holds firm in spite of all disappointments can only be God — God who has loved us and who continues to love us 'to the end.'"

— Pope Benedict XVI, *Spe Salvi*

I am discussing gardening with my mom's roommate at the nursing home. We discover we have a mutual fondness for lavender. "I would love to own a lavender farm!" I exclaim. "We should do it," Irene agrees enthusiastically. Then she adds with a wry chuckle, "Sooner, rather than later." This is a life lesson. We should pursue our dreams sooner, rather than later. And if we can't, we should maintain a positive attitude, like Irene.

June 6

Wait for It

"All things work for good for those who love God."

— Romans 8:28

You've probably heard that expression, "If you want to make God laugh, tell Him your plans." I don't like it. It makes God seem like a vindictive prankster, scoffing at our shy hopes. We used to plan to return to the West Coast. My husband kept up his counseling license in California, and I thought we might live close to my parents in Nevada. I would happily look after them as they grew old, just as my dad had cared for his dad. But things have taken a different turn. God isn't laughing at our plans. He has something better in mind. We just have to wait for it.

JUNE 7

Transforming the Body

"That is Corpus Christi: to celebrate the Eucharist cosmically; to carry it even to our streets and squares so that the world . . . may receive healing and reconciliation."

— Cardinal Joseph Ratzinger, *Images of Hope*

"I believe in the resurrection of the body" we say when we recite the Creed. As our bodies gets old and starts to disintegrate, we may wonder why we would want to drag it around in the afterlife. But, our resurrected bodies will be perfected, glorified, transformed, incorruptible. Because Jesus *is* the Resurrection, and we *become* His body through the Eucharist, we will be raised on the last day. Let's bring the resurrection with us, wherever we go today.

June 8

Battling Demons

"Philothea, since you wish to live a devout life you must not only cease to sin but you must also purify your heart of all affection for sin."

— Saint Francis de Sales, *Introduction to the Devout Life*

When Jesus got out of the boat and stepped into the territory of the Gerasenes (see Mk 5:1-20), He was immediately accosted by a man possessed by a demon. The demoniac threw himself down on his knees and called out to the Son of God. He begged Him not to torture him! How odd and yet how true. Like the demoniac who doesn't want to be cured, we have an odd affection for our pet sins. We are attached to our small vices, those mundane sins (are they really so bad?) that we find hard to give up. We wish God would stop bothering us, demanding things of us, *torturing* us with His constant desire for us to be good! Thank you, Lord, for healing the demoniac anyway, and giving us hope!

June 9

Heart of the Eternal

"For the love of God is broader

than the measure of man's mind;

and the heart of the Eternal

is most wonderfully kind."

— Frederick William Faber, *There's a Wideness in God's Mercy*

When I see my son — whom I clearly remember as a baby — holding *his* son, my grandchild, I am struck by the thought that this must be a tiny glimpse into what eternity is like. For God, every moment is the eternal *now,* eternity in the moment. His loving gaze encompasses everything at once — our past, present, and future.

June 10

Caring for the Caregiver

"Without solitude of heart, our relationships with others easily become needy and greedy, sticky and clinging, dependent and sentimental."

— *Mornings with Henri Nouwen*

A young woman gave up her career to live with her aging father and her mother who had just suffered a massive stroke. She slept on the floor next to her mother's bed, because her mother might need her in the middle of the night. One night, the dutiful daughter burst into tears after the sixth time she was awakened by the insistent bell-ringing. Her mother then reminded her that she had to wake up every two hours to feed her when she was a baby.

Wise spiritual directors tell us there is a difference between humility and being a doormat. Caregivers need to care for themselves, too.

JUNE 11

Paddling to Glory

"Love through pain is a higher form of love. Anybody can love when everything is fine. What's hard about that? Love is proved by sacrifice."

— *Mother Angelica's Private and Pithy Lessons from the Scriptures*

My mom loved watching Mother Angelica on EWTN and had many VHS tapes of the wise and humorous outspoken nun. Now, both my mom and Mother Angelica are in the same boat. Both suffered incapacitating strokes and are unable to speak. I send an email prayer request for my mom to the nuns at Our Lady of the Angels Monastery. Despite suffering great physical pain throughout her entire life, Mother Angelica was always upbeat, joyful, and down-to-earth. Let's hope that we can follow her example.

June 12

Flame of Love

"Abba Lot went to see Abba Joseph and he said to him, 'Abba, as far as I can, I say my little office, I fast a little, I pray and meditate, I live in peace and as far as I can I purify my thoughts. What else can I do?' Then the old man stood up and stretched his hands towards heaven; his fingers became like ten lamps of fire and he said to him, 'If you will, you can become all flame.'"

— *Daily Readings with the Desert Fathers*

Let your love for Christ light you from within.

June 13

Finding Joy

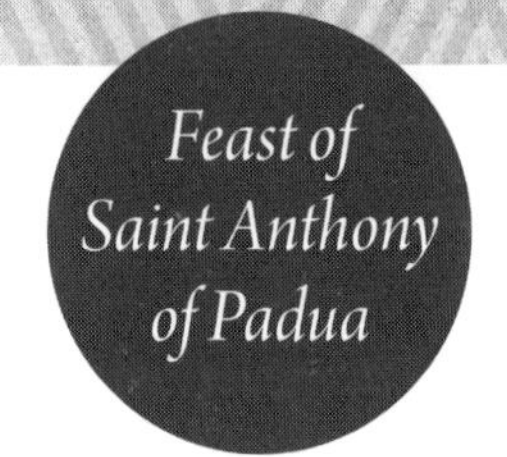

"Happy the misery, then, that leads to better things! And happy darkness, that brings forth light! Those destitute of worldly abundance, like poor people; or of bodily health, like the sick, the blind and the lame — who lack the pleasures of sin — are all the more readily brought into the Lord's supper."

— Saint Anthony of Padua, *Sermon*

Soon after his ordination to the priesthood, Saint Anthony saw the relics of martyred Franciscans. Deeply moved, he decided to join that order and devote himself to spreading the faith in Africa. Instead, he ended up preaching mostly in Europe. It is comforting to know that even a saint changes his mind! The Franciscans were at first unaware of Anthony's intellectual gifts, and he spent his time washing dishes. Providentially, one day at an ordination he was asked to preach spontaneously since no one else had come prepared to speak. His impressive performance took everyone by surprise. From that point on, he was sent out to preach and brought many lost souls back to the faith. Perhaps that is why he is invoked as the finder of lost things! Saint Anthony, pray for us.

June 14

Laying Down the Knife

"'My son,' Abraham answered, 'God himself will provide the sheep for the holocaust.'"

— Genesis 22:8

God tested Abraham up to the very moment when he was about to plunge the knife into his only son's heart. At that breathtaking point — Abraham's knife raised over Isaac tied to the firewood — God said, "Do not lay your hand on the boy." At this moment, we discover that God is indeed a loving father. It must have seemed an eternity to Abraham — and he did not know the outcome, as we do! But, now we know. The time of testing will end, and God will provide everything.

JUNE 15

Lazarus at the Gate

"And lying at his door was a poor man named Lazarus, covered with sores, who would gladly have eaten his fill of the scraps that fell from the rich man's table."

— Luke 16:20-21

Mrs. X. has to pay someone to visit her at the nursing home, because her own children will not. Granted, she is a very difficult character. "What are you looking at?" she grumbles to one resident. "Go back to your room!" she commands lost Mr. Y, who has forgotten where his room is. We all tiptoe past her door, hoping she won't call out for us. There she sits, in her wheelchair, wearing her nightgown and socks, peering around the edge of the door, eyes red-rimmed, waiting to see if someone might come down the hall. She hopes there will be someone who would like to talk to her, because she is lonely. But nobody ever comes just for her.

June 16

People of Faith

"For this reason, I remind you to stir into flame the gift of God."

— 2 Timothy 1:6

Jairus, the synagogue official whose daughter was dying, and the woman suffering from hemorrhages for twelve years were brought together in one Gospel passage (see Mk 5:21-42) for a reason. Both were people of faith. Jairus risked humiliation since he was a synagogue official and probably should have known better than to throw himself at the feet of the itinerant preacher. The woman, too, risked embarrassment in front of the crowd, yet reached out to touch Jesus' cloak. What was their faith like? Was it a hard rock of certainty? Or perhaps they had faith like mine: a tiny flickering flame, glowing warm with hope. It could have been snuffed out with a breath, yet, in fear and trembling, they brought it to Jesus, and it saved them.

June 17

Climbing the Mountain of Time

"I raise my eyes toward the mountains.

From whence shall come my help?"

— Psalm 121:1

We used to sit out on the deck, my dad and I, in comfortable silence. As the evening breeze ruffled the leaves of the locust tree, we listened to the cooing of the doves. We watched the mountains blacken against the cobalt sky, back-lit by the setting sun. My dad spoke less in those days. He had always listened with enthusiasm, relishing the details of our lives, but now he no longer asked questions. He was listening for God's word in his heart, and he was waiting to go back over that mountain, the one he climbed in his youth. And on the other side, beyond the region of thunder, he would find peace.

June 18

Traveling to the Interior

"Sarapion the Sindonite travelled once on a pilgrimage to Rome. Here he was told of a celebrated recluse, a woman who lived always in one small room, never going out. Skeptical about her way of life — for he was himself a great wanderer — Sarapion called on her and asked, 'Why are you sitting here?' To which she replied, 'I am not sitting; I am on a journey.'"

— *Daily Readings with the Desert Fathers*

The bedridden are journeying inward, traveling farther than we can ever know. While we rush about and do many things, those who cannot do, pray. As Jesus tells us, that is the better part.

JUNE 19

Better to Bless

"Do not return evil for evil, or insult for insult; but, on the contrary, a blessing."

— 1 Peter 3:9

Just yesterday, I was on my way to Mass and a driver cut in front of me — and honked at me! I was filled with self-righteous anger because he was in the wrong and didn't even realize it. I wanted to stop and explain the rules of the road to that ignoramus. Then I remembered that I was heading to Mass. Shouldn't I have a more peaceful disposition? As a Christian, shouldn't I pray for that man's soul instead? Offer a blessing, instead of a curse.

June 20

Secret Gift

"Joy is the secret gift of compassion. We keep forgetting it and thoughtlessly look elsewhere."

— Henri Nouwen, *Here and Now*

Henri Nouwen described taking care of a handicapped man named Adam — bathing him, dressing him, brushing his teeth, feeding him. The hours he spent with Adam became his most precious time of the day. One day, a colleague of Nouwen's asked him, "Is this what you got all that education for?" And Nouwen realized that he experienced a greater joy in caregiving than he had ever experienced before in his successful academic career. Joy is the secret gift of compassion.

June 21

What Is It?

"When the layer of dew evaporated, fine flakes were on the surface of the wilderness, fine flakes like hoarfrost on the ground. On seeing it, the Israelites asked one another, 'What is this?' for they did not know what it was. But Moses told them, "It is the bread which the LORD has given you to eat."

— Exodus 16:14-15

The Israelites were grumbling about God, saying they would rather *die* in Egypt with their fleshpots than starve in the wilderness. So God said, "I will rain bread from heaven for you!" And He continued to give us this heavenly bread, daily, like the dewfall. He doesn't whomp us over the head with his sledgehammer, though we often fear that's what He's like. No, He gently offers us His most perfect food: His Son. And we, puzzled, ask, "What is it?" We complain, grumble, and fret. We don't trust that He only wants the greatest happiness for us, that He knows best how to guide us, that He loves us like the best papa.

June 22

Unlocking the Door

"Behold, I have left an open door before you, which no one can close."

— Revelation 3:8

She tried to leave, but the door was locked. She showed me a newsletter from the assisted living facility with photos of happy residents eating lunch at Red Lobster. Why, it had the same name as the place where she lives! Is there perhaps a parallel universe, a facility with the same name, where residents go shopping and out to eat? Yet, here she is, locked in with the ones who cannot speak or walk. There are some whose minds are almost completely gone. I pray that God sends her a companion, a friend or a relative who will take her to Red Lobster.

June 23

The Inventory

"I consider the days of old;

the years long past I remember.

At night I ponder in my heart;

And as I meditate, my spirit probes."

— Psalm 77:6-7

We find my mom's household inventory — twenty-two pages of items single-spaced, including the date the item was purchased and the amount. I wake up in the middle of the night fretting over judgment errors I made sorting through the mountains of stuff. I am a kid again, and I want to ask my dad for his advice. Now I can only offer a prayer of apology and ask for his blessing from heaven. I would need another home if I were to keep everything they owned! Yet, I need nothing larger than my heart to keep the love and memories of my parents alive.

June 24

Humility of Heart

Solemnity of the Nativity of John the Baptist

"He must increase; I must decrease."

— John 3:30

How God treasures every moment of our lives! At the first meeting of Jesus and John, when they were still in their mothers' wombs, John leaped for joy. He recognized his savior, he became a voice in the wilderness, saying "prepare the way of the Lord."

We, too, should be preparing for the coming of the Lord, whether it is His coming into our hearts, or His coming at the end of time. And, to prepare, we must decrease our own selfish desires, our irritations, our list of agenda items. Instead, let the Lord increase. We can do this daily, by thinking less of ourselves and more of the ones we care for.

A Providential Flaw

"O happy fault!"

— *Exsultet*

R.A. Dickey is reviving the knuckleball. When he was with the Mets, the award-winning pitcher won twenty games, the first knuckleballer to do so in decades. Early on, however, things looked bleak for Dickey. After high school, he was a first-round pick with the promise of a large salary, until the doctors discovered he was missing a ligament in his pitching arm. The offer was dropped, and eventually he ended up in the minor leagues.

One day, on a whim, Dickey decided to swim across the rushing, muddy Mississippi River. He nearly drowned. Sobbing, he said his final prayers. Suddenly, he realized that his feet could touch the bottom! Coming out of the river, he was reborn. He started throwing knuckleballs. Out of weakness, comes strength.

June 26

Watered with Love

"It is not the objects of our love that have to be changed; it is our love that has to be changed by being transformed into the love which is the heart of Christ."

— Gerald Vann, O.P., *The Seven Sweet Blessings of Christ*

In days of old, Elisha the prophet purified the water of Jericho, saying "never again shall death or sterility come from it!" (2 Kgs 2:21). In modern times, the Blessed Mother appeared to Saint Bernadette and transformed a humble hidden spring in a poor French town into miraculous, healing waters. I have a tiny bottle of Lourdes water that was a gift. I bring it to my mom, and bless her forehead and her hands. She looks a little surprised, and I don't think it will cure her. But I know it helps.

June 27

Glimpsing Heaven

"If love, even human love, gives so much consolation here, what will love not be in heaven?"

— Saint Josemaría Escrivá, *The Way*

I am wheeling my mom outside when we catch sight of little Nellie under "her" big oak tree. She struggles up from the bench to greet us, determinedly trundling her walker over the uneven grass and tree roots. She greets my mom effusively, though my mom can't answer. "You stopping by makes me so happy," she sighs, though we didn't really stop by, and we weren't very entertaining. Yet, this simple thing, this heartwarming encounter, fills our hearts. Surely, this is a glimpse of His kingdom!

June 28

Faithfulness

"Wherever you go I will go,

wherever you lodge I will lodge.

Your people shall be my people,

and your God, my God."

— Ruth 1:16

When Naomi's husband and her two sons died, she decided to leave the foreign country where she lived and return to Bethlehem, the land of her people. She bid her two daughters-in-law, Orpah and Ruth, farewell. But Ruth begged her mother-in-law, "Do not ask me to abandon or forsake you!" Ruth risked her whole life — the comfort of living in a familiar town, the chance that she would never remarry — to stay, faithful, by Naomi's side. As it turned out, she did remarry, and her son became the father of Jesse, who is the father of King David.

Let's pray that we can be similarly faithful to our relatives, even if we can't know what the future will bring.

JUNE 29

Solemnity of Saints Peter and Paul

Joining the Family

"If you can't preach like Peter, If you can't pray like Paul, Just tell the love of Jesus, And say He died for all."

— *There Is a Balm in Gilead*, hymn

Jesus asked His disciples: "Who do the people say I am?" and "Who do you say that I am?" Pope Emeritus Benedict XVI has said that Jesus was drawing attention to the difference between those who simply know something about Christ (He is a great prophet) and those who are part of His intimate family, the Church. Peter, our first pope, declared, "You are the Messiah, the Son of the living God" (see Luke 9:18-20). It is at this critical juncture that His friends had to choose to follow Him. This choice involved intimacy, but also risk. Are we willing to be part of His family, the Church? Or, do we want to keep a safe distance?

June 30

Holiness Is Where You Find It

"For a single cup of water God has promised to his faithful a sea of perfect bliss."

— Saint Francis de Sales, *Introduction to the Devout Life*

Saint Francis de Sales originally wrote his letters about the devout life to Madame de Charmoisy, the wife of a relative, to whom he was giving spiritual direction. He told her that even if God did not ask a dramatic martyrdom ("does not demand your eyes of you") you can give Him something small. It can be a bad cold, a grumpy husband, a lost ring, a feeling of embarrassment. Any of these small trials, if accepted lovingly, are highly pleasing. And you, dear caregiver, whatever you do today for your loved one, you are immensely pleasing to God.

July 1

The Weight of Joy

"Being patient. . . . This does not mean being sad. No, no, it's another thing! This means bearing, carrying the weight of difficulties, the weight of contradictions, the weight of tribulations on our shoulders. This Christian attitude of bearing up: of being patient."

— Pope Francis, *Homily,* May 7, 2013

Being joyful while carrying a burden: This is indeed a virtue. Both caregivers and those cared for can pray together for the grace of being patient.

July 2

Attending the Meek

"O Lord, you will hear the desire of the meek;

you will strengthen their heart, you will incline your ear."

— Psalm 10:17, NRSVCE

There is a beautiful Asian woman at the nursing home who seems oblivious to her surroundings. Sometimes, she falls forward at dinner, her head resting on the table where she sits. The nurses and attendants just leave her there. I notice that she always has her hair and nails done. Someone loves her and cares for her. One day, I meet her daughter! I tell her, "Your mom is so beautiful!" The elderly woman's lips move, but she speaks so softly that I hear nothing. Her daughter tells me, "She says thank you."

July 3

Touching the Wound

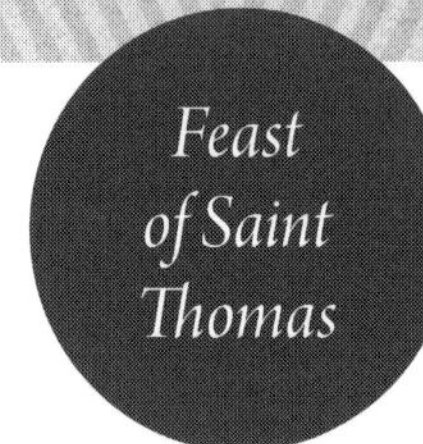

"Some people believe straightaway, such as Mary Magdalene. Others believe after a period of doubt. And others need to put their finger in the wound, like Thomas. Each individual has his own way of coming to believe. Faith is the encounter with Jesus Christ."

— Pope Francis, *Conversations with Jorge Bergoglio: His Life in His Own Words*

Our faith respects the body; it is very physical, real. Mary wept and dried Jesus' feet with her hair. Thomas stuck his hand into Jesus' wounds. Jesus healed the blind man using spit and mud. Jesus knew what it is to doubt (and how anxiety can be felt physically). He knew how best to reassure us. Sometimes we need to touch the wound. Physical touch is so important — a big hug, a clasp of the hand, a foot massage, a kiss.

July 4

Breaking the Prison Walls

"I tried to smile. I struggled to raise my hand. I could not. I felt nothing, not the slightest spark of warmth or charity. And so again I breathed a silent prayer. Jesus, I cannot forgive him. Give me Your forgiveness."

— Corrie Ten Boom, *The Hiding Place*

How was it possible for Corrie Ten Boom to forgive the SS officer who had held her captive in the concentration camp, who had ruthlessly mocked the starving, suffering prisoners? Yet, with God's help, she did forgive him, and she went around the world speaking God's message of healing. Forgiveness breaks the prison walls of our own bitterness and past wounds. It frees us to step into the light and joy of God's love. We don't have to *feel* as though we love those who have hurt us; we just need to want to. Ask Jesus to help you forgive.

JULY 5

Worry

"Learn then that I, I alone, am God,

and there is no god beside me.

It is I who bring both death and life."

— Deuteronomy 32:39, NAB

I never thought about my own death until my father passed away and my mom became incapacitated as a result of a massive stroke. Now I worry. Who will take care of my mom if I die? I'm the only one who understands her finances, knows her medical history and where she keeps the key to the safety-deposit box. I pay her bills, keep tabs on the maintenance of her home, and manage her health care. Some days, these details overwhelm me. At these times, I throw my hands up and say, "Lord, you've got this." Worry happens when I try to solve all the problems of life myself, using my own ingenuity and effort, forgetting that God is in charge.

July 6

Mighty Deeds

"Many will say to me on that day, 'Lord, Lord, did we not prophesy in your name? Did we not drive out demons in your name? Did we not do mighty deeds in your name?' Then I will declare to them solemnly, 'I never knew you. Depart from me, you evildoers.'"

— Matthew 7:22-23

How astonished these mighty deed workers will be when they discover that, although they did great things for Jesus, they are not saved. Christ doesn't want impressive deeds. He wants us to do God's will. And His will may be something very simple, unimpressive to the world. It may be caring for an elderly parent or a sick child. It may simply be doing your daily tasks with love.

JULY 7

Shared Suffering

"Indeed, to accept the 'other' who suffers, means that I take up his suffering in such a way that it becomes mine also. Because it has now become a shared suffering, though, in which another person is present, this suffering is penetrated by the light of love."

— Pope Benedict XVI, *Spe Salvi*

We wish that we could bear some of the pain of our suffering friends. And yet, in a sense, we do. In caregiving, we take a little of our loved one's pain into our hearts, onto our shoulders. Simply by being there, by accepting the work of a caregiver — the inconveniences, the humiliations, the dreariness of the daily duties, the worries — you bring Christ's love to the one for whom you care. You share in the suffering.

July 8

Beautiful Mercy

"We need to understand properly this mercy of God, this merciful Father who is so patient. . . . Let us remember the Prophet Isaiah who says that even if our sins were scarlet, God's love would make them white as snow. This mercy is beautiful!"

— Pope Francis, *Angelus,* March 17, 2013

Jonah was a cranky prophet. He prophesied the destruction of the evil city of Nineveh. But, when the entire city repented and did penance for their sins, God forgave them. Jonah, however, was still angry. He wanted to see the city punished.

God is merciful, unlike us! We hold onto our anger, our bitterness, our memories of slights big and small. So, God took away Jonah's gourd plant in order to teach him a lesson about mercy. Sometimes, our sufferings are lessons in mercy.

July 9

Comfort-givers

"They give and they listen, they see the spark of life wherever it is and fan it by the warm breath of their humanity; they reverence the solitude of other people's souls; they bear other people's burdens and rejoice in their joy, without imposing upon them. Not only do they tread delicately not to crush the broken reed, but they go down on their knees to bind it up. They take the neglected Christ Child to their own hearts instinctively and comfort him."

— Caryll Houselander, *The Passion of the Infant Christ*

You are a caregiver: you comfort the infant Christ.

July 10

Be on the Lookout

"That is the religious experience: the astonishment of meeting someone who has been waiting for you all along. From that moment on, for me, God is the One who te primerea — 'springs it on you.' You search for Him, but He searches for you first. You want to find Him, but He finds you first."

— Pope Francis, *Conversations with Jorge Bergoglio: His Life in His Own Words*

You have to be on the lookout, though. Would you even realize who it is, if you're not? He doesn't look the way you might expect Him to look, the almighty God. Why, He's the lonely elderly woman sitting on her bench in the sun, wishing someone would stop by just for her. Or, He's the Latino gardener who planted all the tulip bulbs. He's the janitor who offers me a blessing. Or, He's the small piece of unleavened bread.

July 11

Hemmed in on All Sides

"But he passed through the midst of them and went away."

— Luke 4:30

Jesus is surrounded by an enraged mob that tries to hurl Him over a cliff. Yet, He passes right through them. Sometimes, we feel as though we are surrounded on all sides by irrational situations, angry people, insurmountable problems. Yet, if we just take hold of Jesus, follow Him, we can pass right through the midst of them.

July 12

Blessing the Song of the World

"You are called, with all the saints, to bless in the power of Christ's priesthood the song of the world, and to perfect it."

— Gerald Vann, O.P., *The Seven Sweet Blessings of Christ*

A blind opera singer comes to perform for the elderly at the nursing home. His voice is powerful yet gentle, too, bringing tears to our eyes. At the end, I wheel my mom up to him, to thank him. He can't see her, and she can't speak, but she holds her hand out to him, and I guide his hand to hers. Two souls, each suffering in their own way, each with a blessing to give.

JULY 13

Light of Love

"The light of faith is unique, since it is capable of illuminating every aspect of human existence. A light this powerful cannot come from ourselves but from a more primordial source: in a word, it must come from God. Faith is born of an encounter with the living God who calls us and reveals his love, a love which precedes us and upon which we can lean for security and for building our lives."

— Pope Francis, *Lumen Fidei*

In Plato's allegory of the cave, we are prisoners chained in a dark den lit only by the light of a fire which casts shadows on the wall. We take these shadows for reality because we've never been outside the cave. One day, when we emerge from the cave of this world into the light of the Son, we will be astounded by reality. All will be unveiled: "Nothing is concealed that will not be revealed, nor secret that will not be known" (Mt 10:26). And nothing you do in secret and out of kindness will be unrewarded.

July 14

Honor Your Father

"Those who honor their father will have joy in their own children,
and when they pray they will be heard."

— Sirach 3:5, NRSVCE

Just before he died, Tobit called his son to him and told him to flee the city, because the destruction of Nineveh that had been foretold would surely come to pass. Tobiah obeyed his father and left Nineveh to live with his aging father-in-law and mother-in-law, taking respectful care of them until their deaths (see Tb 14:13). Tobiah didn't dismiss his father's claims (as we might) as the ravings of a senile, old man. What a beautiful example!

July 15

The Power of a Look

"He leaped up, stood, and walked around, and went into the temple with them, walking and jumping and praising God."

— Acts 3:8

The man referred to in the above passage was crippled from birth and sat every day at the Beautiful Gate of the Temple, begging. Peter and John said to him, "Look at us!" They commanded him to rise up and walk. He did better: he was jumping and leaping, dancing and praising God. The nursing assistant tells my mom, "Look at me." She looks. He asks her where she is having pain, but she cannot tell us. He says that he will help her, and she trusts him.

JULY 16

You vs. the World

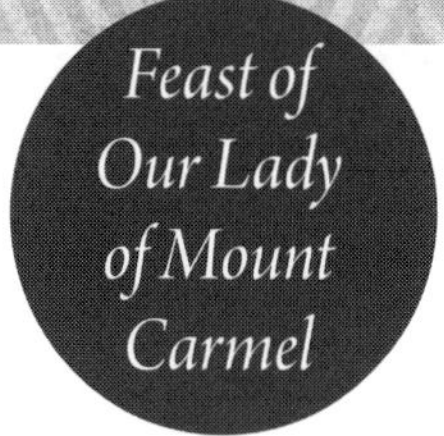

"Answer me, LORD! Answer me, that this people may know that you, LORD, are God and that you have turned their hearts back to you."

— 1 Kings 18:37

It was on Mount Carmel that Elijah, a lone prophet speaking out against 450 false prophets, proved that the Lord is the one, true God. Does it sometimes feel as though it's you against the world? On this date in the year 1251, Our Lady appeared to Saint Simon Stock, giving him the brown scapular. She said that it would be a protection in danger, a pledge of peace: "Whosoever dies wearing this scapular shall not suffer eternal fire."

When you feel outnumbered, surrounded by voices of negativity and gloom, when it's you against all the naysayers, turn to Our Lady. She will bring you peace and protection.

July 17

Never Alone

"What would happen if we all started asking one another for help — if we found the humility to turn to one another and say, 'I can't do this on my own; I need you. Please help me!'? We would, in time, find ourselves inside a mysterious and wonderful experience: real human community."

— John Janaro, *Never Give Up*

How often does it happen that when we are feeling particularly stressed or burdened or suffering, we try to solve our problems alone. Like sick animals, we crawl into a cave to lick our wounds. Yet the real solution is exactly the opposite. We need to share our troubles, bring our problems to the light of day, seek out our good friends and ask for help. We are part of a community, the Body of Christ. And praying before the Blessed Sacrament, we discover we are never alone.

Feast of Saint Camillus de Lellis

July 18

Compassionate Love

"As a person grows in virtue, his love becomes compassionate and caring, with heartfelt tenderness. Love, thus felt, adds something rich to our care for others, even our enemies. Such was the compassionate love of Christ."

— Emmerich Vogt, *The Freedom to Love*

Saint Camillus de Lellis was a hot-tempered soldier and a gambler before he became a saint. A big man (about six foot six) with a tendency to get into fights, he left home at seventeen for a military career. Soon, he developed a serious leg ailment that plagued him for the rest of his life. By the time he was twenty-four, he had gambled away everything he owned, even his clothes. Destitute and unable to find work, he repented for his former life. He devoted himself to caring for the sick. After discovering the deplorable state of hospitals of the time, he vowed to reform them. Eventually, under the direction of Saint Philip Neri, he became a priest and founded the Servants of the Sick to care for those afflicted by the plague and other serious illnesses.

July 19

Healing the Paralyzed

"'Lord, my servant is lying at home paralyzed, suffering dreadfully.' He said to him, 'I will come and cure him.'"

— Matthew 8:6

During the very early days of the Church, when it was just being built up (see Acts 9:31-34), Peter met a man named Aeneas, who had been confined to bed for eight years, paralyzed. Peter told him: "Jesus Christ heals you, get up and make your bed."

Your loving and healing touch raises the spirits of those who are confined to bed. This is a miracle, too.

July 20

Reflections of God

"The great spiritual challenge is to discover, over time, that the limited, conditional, and temporal love we receive from parents, husbands, wives, children, teachers, colleagues and friends are reflections of the unlimited, unconditional, and everlasting love of God."

— Henri Nouwen, *Here and Now*

Heath White is a military man, top gun pilot, and marathon runner. He put pressure on his wife to have an abortion when they discovered their child had Down syndrome and would not, therefore, be perfect. He ended up discovering how truly wonderful his daughter was, and had to rethink his understanding of perfection. He finally realized that his love for her was perfect. He was not perfect, she was not perfect, but his love for her was perfect.

July 21

Family Therapy

"[Tobiah] then departed with his wife and children for Media, where he settled in Ecbatana with his father-in-law Raguel. He took respectful care of his aging father-in-law and mother-in-law."

— Tobit 14:12-13

My friend's father-in-law became terribly ill at age eighty-seven and was confined to a wheelchair. The whole family decided to move in with him to keep an eye on Dad. This necessitated a massive renovation of his home to provide a separate studio. During the process of renovating, their father suddenly perked up. He no longer needed a wheelchair or even a walker. Robin asked, "Are you sure you still want five people to move in here with you?" He pondered the matter carefully and thoughtfully replied, "Well, I'm bound to get old *eventually*, so I'd rather have you here when it happens."

For five years now they have all been living happily (and injury free) together. Dad hasn't gotten old yet!

July 22

Feast of Saint Mary Magdalene

Eye on the Prize

"When he had risen, early on the first day of the week, he appeared first to Mary Magdalene, out of whom he had driven seven demons."

— Mark 16:9

A painting of Mary Magdalene by Georges de La Tour shows a young, beautiful Mary sitting at a table gazing into the flame of a candle, a skull on her lap. She loved Jesus when He was in the flesh. He freed her from seven demons. She stayed by Him at the foot of the Cross. And now her love for Jesus was enflamed by her reading of Scripture. Yet, she is also very sensual, with her long hair loose, her blouse draped low, and her skirt pulled up showing her bare legs. Perhaps de La Tour wanted to remind us that, despite our own earthiness and our attraction to the beauty of the world, we must keep our eyes fixed on the flame of love that is Christ in our hearts.

July 23

Feast of Saint Bridget

Faithful Care

"You allowed your most holy mother to suffer so much, even though she had never sinned nor ever even consented to the smallest sin. Humbly you looked down upon her with your gentle loving eyes, and to comfort her you entrusted her to the faithful care of your disciple."

— Prayer attributed to Saint Bridget, Office of Readings for July 23

On those days when I struggle to understand why my mom must suffer so much, without relief, and seemingly without reason, I can pray as Saint Bridget prayed: "*even your most holy mother was allowed to suffer.*" And in the very moment of her deepest grief and suffering, the Blessed Mother was entrusted to the disciple whom Jesus loved. Jesus holds caregivers in a special place in His heart for He entrusted His own suffering mother to the gentle care of His beloved disciple.

July 24

What Is More Real?

"In the Eucharist we learn to see the heights and depths of reality. The bread and wine are changed into the body and blood of Christ, who becomes present in his passover to the Father: this movement draws us, body and soul, into the movement of all creation towards its fulfillment in God."

— Pope Francis, *Lumen Fidei*

I am listening to an interview with a man who has been dubbed the "father of virtual reality." He cautions us about spending too much time with technology. Reality is being mediated by software, by the Internet, and the "siren servers," he says. It occurs to me that as our actions center more and more on the virtual sphere (our daily interactions with Facebook, Twitter and other social media), we simultaneously become less capable of seeing what lies beneath appearances, of experiencing the *ground* of being, or of intuiting what is *more* real. In the Eucharist, we experience the heights and depths of reality. We receive Jesus himself in the mystery of faith, the mystery upholding all reality.

JULY 25

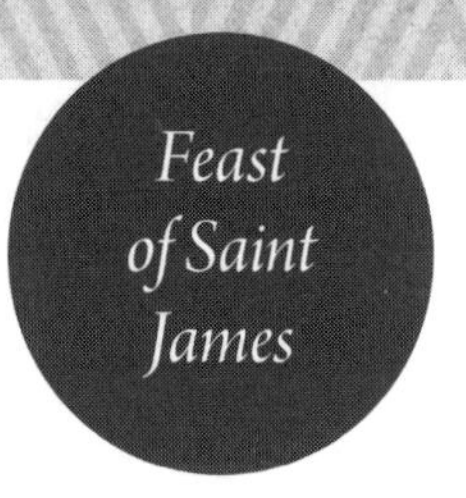

A Big Personality

"He called them. Immediately they left the boat and their father, and followed him."

—Matthew 4:21-22, NRSVCE

The painting of Saint James by Peter Paul Rubens shows a handsome, strong man with thick, black, curly hair and a full-sized, mountain-man beard. He looks out directly at the viewer, a little pugnaciously. After all, James, son of Zebedee, was nicknamed by Jesus as one of the Sons of Thunder. James wanted to call down fire and destruction on a town that didn't welcome Christ, and he also asked to sit at Christ's right hand when he was in his glory. Audacious, perhaps. A big personality with a temper. But when Jesus called him, he immediately followed.

Sometimes, we can be audacious, too, in our requests. And, sometimes, we get angry. God wants us to be real with Him.

July 26

Carrying Christ

"You, who are not prisoners, who are not held in one place, go often to Holy Communion. Carry Christ everywhere in your hearts. Make your souls monstrances, and go into those places where Our Lord has never been adored in the Host, where the monstrance has never been lifted up."

— Caryll Houselander, *The Passion of the Infant Christ*

Houselander is quoting an anonymous priest who was imprisoned and eventually killed for his faith. His hands had been cut off so he could never offer Mass again. Think of the many unknown martyrs of our time and of all those who suffer for the faith — imprisoned priests, those who oppose forced abortions in China, the Christian slaves of Somalia, and many more. We are asked to do only a simple thing: to receive Our Lord in Communion. We should visit those who are imprisoned by their beds, the four walls of the nursing home, and their illness.

July 27

Seeing Both Sides

"At every moment of our life we have an opportunity to choose joy. . . . We always have a choice to live the moment as a cause for resentment or as a cause for joy."

— Henri Nouwen, *Here and Now*

God always grants a special grace whenever he calls someone to a special vocation. Of course, we know this is true for priests and nuns. But, it's also true for spouses, parents, and caregivers. God gives us every gift of the Holy Spirit necessary to accomplish the task at hand. Sometimes, we make it hard on ourselves when we worry and complain and feel resentful and burdened. Instead, relax! Let this moment be a cause for joy.

July 28

Return on Investment

"Jesus said, 'Amen, I say to you, there is no one who has given up house or brothers or sisters or mother or father or children or lands for my sake and for the sake of the gospel who will not receive a hundred times more now in this present age: houses and brothers and sisters and mothers and children and lands, with persecutions, and eternal life in the age to come.'"

— Mark 10:29-30

Writer Sheldon Vanauken's beloved wife, Davy, died prematurely at age forty. Just one year prior, without her husband's knowledge, she had offered her life for his conversion. How many of those who are in the nursing home or shut in, or confined to their sickbeds, are silently, secretly offering their sufferings, their illnesses, for the sake of their loved ones? They — and you who care for them — will be blessed a hundredfold.

JULY 29

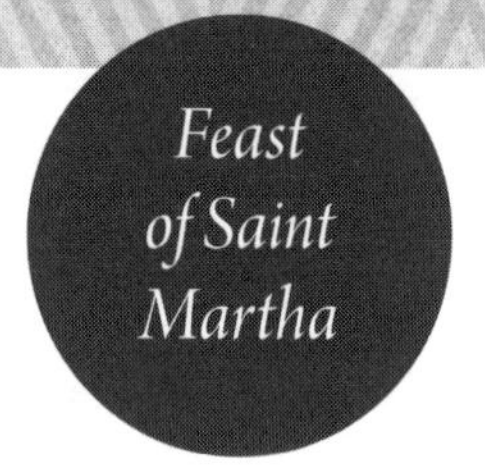

First Things First

"Jesus does not, of course, blame Martha's work, but only her worrying about it."

— Saint Thérèse of Lisieux, *The Story of a Soul*

Don't we all relate to Martha? She is all about her work. She's efficient, she gets things done. When Lazarus was ill, near death, she sent away for Jesus. When He finally showed up, she marched up to Him and called Him out for not coming sooner. Then, when Mary is sitting at Jesus' feet, she complains, "Tell her to help me!"

When we are feeling swamped by our many responsibilities, worrying about our long list of things to do, our anxiety can obscure the face of Jesus. Let's recall that Christ wants for us the "better part." We should put our time with Christ, our prayer, first.

July 30

Sharing the Good News

"Is there not a day or even an hour in which we could not give a tear or a smile to someone who is suffering? Cannot a word from us strengthen a soul in distress? Cannot an act of pure love coming from the depths of ourselves brighten a sad life?"

— Elizabeth Leseur, *My Spirit Rejoices*

Mrs. X. is in rare form today. She's mocking the patients with memory problems and cursing the nursing assistants. Her eyes are hard, her mouth in a spiteful twist. "Hi, Mrs. X.!" I say, cheerily. "Go see your momma," she grumbles. Can you blame her for her fury, when she's been left alone to die? Who will bring her the good news that God loves her and will never abandon her?

July 31

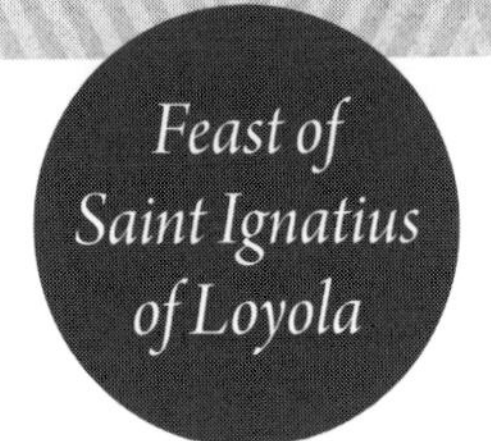

Turning Point

"The greatest consolation he received was to look at the sky and the stars, which he often did and for a long time, because as a result he felt within himself a very great desire to serve Our Lord. He often thought about his intention and wished to be healed completely now so he could take the road."

— *The Autobiography of Saint Ignatius Loyola*

A young, headstrong Basque soldier named Inigo de Loyola, was seriously injured in both legs during the Battle of Pamplona. He was sent to his family's castle to recover. During his painful convalescence, he was given religious books to read rather than the popular romances that he preferred. This was the turning point of his life. He discovered that when he read about vain and worldly pursuits inspired by his books of chivalry, he did not experience the peace and happiness that accompanied his reading and imagining the lives of the saints.

We can act in this same spirit. We can talk to the sick about Christ, His life, and the lives of the saints. Pray together a decade of the Rosary. You, and perhaps those you care for, will experience the same peace and joy that Saint Ignatius did.

August 1

Gifted

"Do not bury your talents! Set your stakes on great ideals, the ideals that enlarge the heart, the ideals of service that make your talents fruitful. Life is not given to us to be jealously guarded for ourselves, but is given to us so that we may give it in turn."

— Pope Francis, *General Audience,* April 24, 2013

Joseph of the Old Testament had an unusual talent. He had crazy dreams and the gift of interpreting dreams, like some Jungian guru. His brothers taunted him: "*Here comes that master dreamer!*" Yet this curious gift makes him invaluable to Pharaoh and ultimately saves his life and that of his whole family. Do you have an unusual or seemingly insignificant talent? Thank God for this gift. It is a blessing for you and your loved ones.

August 2

Other Worlds

"'But do you really mean, Sir,' said Peter, 'that there could be other worlds — all over the place, just around the corner — like that?' 'Nothing is more probable,' said the Professor."

— C.S. Lewis, *The Lion, the Witch and the Wardrobe*

Fairy tales frequently have characters who are not what they appear:. For example, the ugly frog is really a prince, the swan maiden is under a spell, the fox is a cunning advisor, the river is a magical river. How much of what (and who) we encounter each day is not what it seems, or is perhaps Someone in disguise? Saints and Scripture (and some fairy tales!) caution us to treat everyone we meet with the utmost dignity and care, as if the person is Jesus in disguise.

August 3

The Host Life

"The Host life may be lived . . . in people who have to be wheeled about, washed, dressed, and undressed by others; who are literally obliged to offer themselves to God in the hands of other people, like the Host in the priest's hands at the Mass."

— Caryll Houselander, *The Reed of God*

Every day, in tabernacles across the earth, Jesus rests, silent, waiting. This is the eternal God, waiting for you and me to come visit Him. Here, in the tabernacle, He does not go out to us. He waits for us to come to Him. Just as the father of the prodigal son waited at his window, as Dr. Lillian waits on the bench, and my mom waits in her bed, God is helpless. He is unable to move without hands to lift Him up. Silent, never forcing himself on us, but thrilled — *thrilled* — when we (so unworthily) merely pay a visit.

August 4

Mary Our Mother

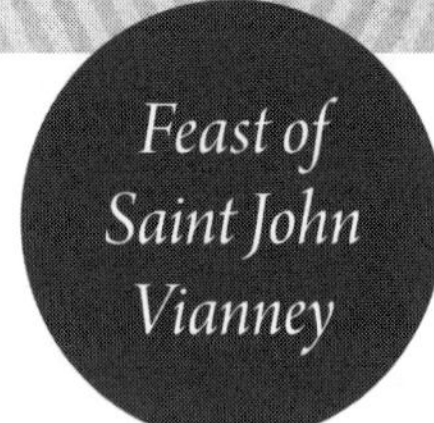

"When we pray properly, sorrows disappear like snow before the sun."

— Saint John Vianney, *Catechetical Instructions*

We've all heard about pious men and women who die peacefully, holding their rosary beads. My mom loved the Rosary and prayed it daily. Now, it hangs on the feeding tube, just out of reach. I take it down, and we will say a decade together, though she has lost the words. Our Blessed Mother understands, and she will wrap her loving arms around my mom and console her, just as she held her only child after the Crucifixion.

There are those who suffer daily upon the cross of pain and loneliness and exhaustion. We pray that their sorrows will melt away like snow before the sun.

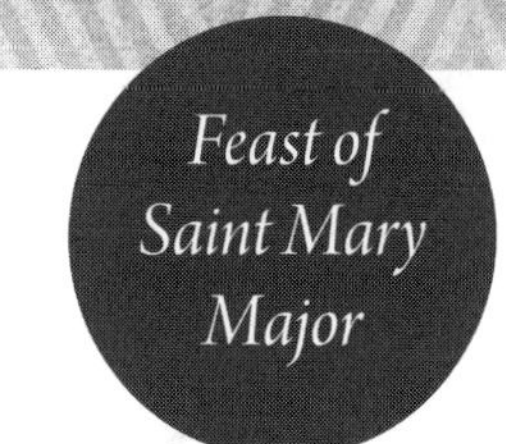

August 5

Resting in the House of God

"The still regions of the soul that otherwise would be pushed aside by the pressures of cares and routine become free when we entrust ourselves to the rhythm of this house of God."

— Cardinal Joseph Ratzinger, *Images of Hope*

It is said that a miraculous snowfall occurred during a hot August night many centuries ago, marking the spot where Rome's Basilica of Saint Mary Major was to be built. An ancient image of the Blessed Mother, gently clasping the child Jesus in both hands, rests here. Pope Saint Gregory the Great carried the image, *Salus Populi Romani*, through the streets of Rome during the Black Plague, and the city was miraculously freed from the pestilence.

Pope Benedict XVI writes that we cannot fail to be consoled when we see how God looks out through the kindly eyes of the Blessed Mother, to heal and protect us.

August 6

Feast of the Transfiguration of the Lord

Things Hidden

"Behold, I make all things new."

— Revelation 21:5

Our Lord in the Blessed Sacrament has chosen to hide himself in this way. Similarly, His divinity was hidden when He walked the earth as a man. But at the Transfiguration, the veil was slightly lifted, revealing His dazzling appearance. In the adoration chapel, the white host is surrounded by gold and shimmering jewels. It reminds us of the possibility of transfiguration. How much else is hidden, veiled, on this earth? Gnarled fingers, silent lips, broken bodies waiting to be transfigured.

AUGUST 7

Sacred Chrism

"You signed her with the sign of the cross of Jesus . . . and under that sign your love will grow deeper and wider even when your heart is pierced."

— Henri Nouwen, *Here and Now*

Father (the one who drives a bright yellow jeep) anoints my mom's forehead and hands with sacred chrism. Saint Francis de Sales writes that sacred chrism is made up of olive oil representing Christ's meekness, and balm representing His humility. The sick and dying need these two virtues for their final journey. But so, too, do caregivers! We should have meekness in dealing with the daily duties, often small and unrecognized, and sometimes met with rebukes or anger. We need humility in placing ourselves at the service of another.

August 8

You Can't Do It All

"Our mission in this life is not perfection, but holiness. God doesn't want you to feel guilty because you can't do it all."

— Mother Angelica, *Answers, Not Promises*

As long as Moses kept his hands up, Israel prevailed in the battle against Amalek. When he let his hands rest, Amalek prevailed. But Moses grew tired. So, "Aaron and Hur supported his hands, one on one side and one on the other, so that his hands remained steady until sunset" (Ex 17:12). Sometimes, we need help caring for our loved ones.

August 9

Who Wishes to Enter?

"Behold, I stand at the door and knock. If anyone hears my voice and opens the door, [then] I will enter his house and dine with him, and he with me."

— Revelation 3:20

Majid knocks on the door, and my mom is thrilled to see him. He is a long-lost cousin, or Lazarus himself, raised from the dead! He smiles a wide, toothy smile and says in his elegant accent, "Don't worry, I am here!" I had been trying to figure out for an hour what was bothering my mom, but he enters and all is well.

When we open our hearts and allow Christ to enter, He will fill us with his peace.

August 10

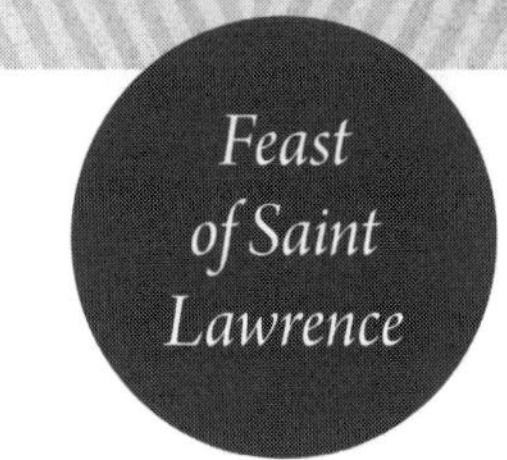

Richer than You Imagine

"The kingdom of heaven is like a treasure buried in a field, which a person finds and hides again, and out of joy goes and sells all that he has and buys that field."

— Matthew 13:44

In the year 258, when Emperor Valerian was persecuting the Church, he commanded Saint Lawrence, a deacon, to bring him the treasure of the Church. Lawrence brought him all the poor, crippled, and diseased people of Rome. Lawrence said, "These are the true treasures of the Church." Though she can no longer speak or walk, my mom is a temple of the Holy Spirit, and my true treasure.

August 11

Here Comes the Son!

"In the morning let me hear of your mercy,

for in you I trust."

— Psalm 143:8

I watch the sun rise. The glowing orb presses upward against the darkness, and the night gives way to a gold and lavender sky, just like a Maxfield Parrish painting.

God gives us this metaphor of himself, written on the morning. Each day, His light pushes away the darkness of our sin, our failures, our sadness. We begin each day with new hope.

August 12

Crankiness

"If we wait for some people to become agreeable or attractive before we begin to love them, we will never begin."

— Thomas Merton, *No Man Is an Island*

Elderly people can sometimes be very cranky. A group of small boys was taunting the Old Testament prophet Elisha, calling him names: "baldhead, baldhead!" The prophet summoned some she-bears who ripped the boys to shreds. Not a gentle old man.

Saints were cranky, too. Saint Jerome, for example, was famously grumpy and ill-tempered. This reminds me that we all are beloved by God: cranky and sweet, ugly and beautiful, enemy and friend alike. God calls each one of us to himself, and to eternal life.

AUGUST 13

Full Comfort

"I will heal them.

I will lead them and restore full comfort to them

and to those who mourn for them."

— Isaiah 57:18

The nursing assistants come every two hours to change my mom's position. They are very attentive to her slightest possible discomfort since she cannot move herself. God assures us that He will heal us, and more. He will give us full comfort. Not just a little comfort, mind you — not just a pat on the back or a passing platitude — but *full* comfort. There will be comfort not only to those who are in need of healing, but also for those who mourn for them! So, full comfort for both my mom and me. The promise itself is comforting!

August 14

I Will Go for You

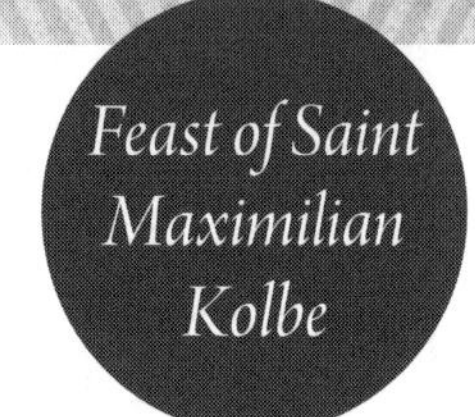

"No one has greater love than this, to lay down one's life for one's friends."

— John 15:13

When Saint Maximilian Kolbe was a child, he had a vision of the Blessed Mother offering him one of two crowns: he could choose either purity or martyrdom. He told her that he would accept both. Maximilian Kolbe became a Franciscan priest and founded the Crusade of Mary Immaculate, publishing the very popular monthly periodical, *Knight of the Immaculate*. In 1941, he drew the attention of the Gestapo and was arrested. As the police drove up to his monastery, he exclaimed, "Praised be Jesus Christ," and willingly entered into His passion. He was sent to Auschwitz, where he prayed with the dying, gave away his own shares of bread, and finally, offered to take the place of a condemned prisoner.

While they do not trade places as Saint Maximilian Kolbe did, caregives share by their compassionate care in the "passion" of their loved ones.

AUGUST 15

Solemnity of the Assumption of the Blessed Virgin Mary

Be Filled with Love

"[Mary] is intimately united to her Risen Son,
the Victor over sin and death, fully conformed to him.
But the Assumption is a reality that touches us too, for it points us in a luminous way toward our destiny, that of humanity and of history. In Mary, indeed, we contemplate that reality of glory to which each one of us and the entire Church is called."

— Pope Benedict XVI, *Angelus, Solemnity of the Assumption of the Blessed Virgin Mary,* August 15, 2012

Mary is assumed, body and soul, into heaven. What does this mean for us, who struggle daily with our physical bodies, with our fear of death and dying? How does it help to ponder this mystery of Our Lady? Mary is so completely filled with grace, with the love of Jesus and the Father, that she, like Christ, overcomes death. And what is resurrection but the power of love over death? (There wasn't even a little bit of her, not one fiber or molecule, that wasn't love.) And so she goes straight to heaven, bypassing the grave.

What this means for us today, with our swollen joints or aching back, our fear of pain and abandonment, is that the more we strive to fill ourselves with love, the closer we will be to heaven.

August 16

Abundant Life

"I came so that they might have life and have it more abundantly. I am the good shepherd. A good shepherd lays down his life for the sheep."

— John 10:10-11

Jesus tells us He is the gate for the sheep. Whoever enters through Him will be saved (see Jn 10:7). The sheep can go in and come out and have pasture. There, they have safety, food, tender care by the Good Shepherd himself.

My grandfather was a sheepherder. He was a *good* sheepherder. His sheep were fat and never mangy looking, like some other ranchers' sheep. And he knew his sheep. From a great distance he could spot one of his own sheep that strayed into a neighboring ranch. Jesus is both gate and shepherd, and He offers us not only life, but an *abundant* life.

August 17

Our Father's Love

"We are not the sum of our weaknesses and failures, we are the sum of the Father's love for us and our real capacity to become the image of His Son Jesus."

— Saint John Paul II, *World Youth Day,* Toronto, 2002

God the Father does not judge us. Jesus shows us His Father, using the parable of the prodigal son. The father gives his rebellious son his entire inheritance. He knows his son will squander the money, but he lets him have it anyway. Then, he waits for him at the window, his heart heavy with longing. He peers down the road and hopes to see his son return. His heart leaps as he catches sight of his son when he is still far off, way down the road. The dusty and emaciated traveler's shoulders are drooping, but the father knows his son's walk. He can spot him even at a distance! And then he throws a party.

"Nor does the Father judge anyone, but he has given all judgment to his Son" (Jn 5:22). What kind of father is this, who judges no one?

AUGUST 18

Payback

"The rewards of compassion are not things to wait for. They are hidden in compassion itself."

— Henri Nouwen, *Here and Now*

Notice the people at the shopping mall or at the gym. Are they happy, serene? Or, do many seem anxious, self-absorbed? At the assisted living facility, the employees greet us cheerfully, taking their time to ask how we are, or they simply comment on the beautiful weather. They are happy to be here. They know that this is where they should be, where they can make a difference. They feel the rewards of compassion.

August 19

Window to Heaven

"Much on earth is hidden from us, but to make up for that we have been given a precious mystic sense of our living bond with the other world, with the higher heavenly world, and the roots of our thoughts and feelings are not here but in other worlds."

— Fyodor Dostoyevsky, *The Brothers Karamazov*

It is said that the first icon was not created by human hands. Legend has it that as Jesus was on His final journey to Jerusalem, King Abgar of Edessa, who was ill with leprosy, sent for Him. Instead, Jesus sent an image of His face, imprinted on a piece of linen. This image miraculously healed the king.

My mom has an icon — *Pantocrator*, an image of Christ the Almighty — that I've brought from her house to mine. His eyes are serious, but not angry, representing both His justice and mercy. He holds the Bible in His hands, telling us that to read it is to discover Him. There are no shadows in icons because all bodies are glorified, dwelling in the eternal light of God. This icon may not be miraculous, but it invites us to silent contemplation. We can attain, for a moment, a glimpse of other worlds.

August 20

The Visit

"And how does this happen to me, that the mother of my Lord should come to me?"

— Luke 1:43

How is it that when Mary greets Elizabeth, Elizabeth knows that she is in the presence of God? Elizabeth is aware of this Presence — "the mother of my Lord" has come to visit — even though this Presence is hidden within Mary's womb. Jesus is also hidden daily in the Host. And He is hidden in the one who cannot speak or move, lying in bed, waiting for someone to visit.

Hidden in you, the one who visits.

August 21

Resurrection

"Jacob lived in the land of Egypt for seventeen years. 'When I lie down with my ancestors, take me out of Egypt and bury me in their burial place.'"

— Genesis 47:28,30

The cicadas lay hidden underground for seventeen years. All at once, in a huge multitude, they rise from their burial grounds, resplendent in their shimmery translucent skins, singing and buzzing in grand synchronicity. For seventeen years, they wait silently. Then, resurrection. Some of the residents of the nursing home have lived there for more than a decade. They are, in a way, buried. Waiting to rise one day, shimmering and singing.

August 22

Cinderella

"What is man that you are mindful of him,

or the son of man that you care for him?

You made him for a little while lower than the angels."

— Hebrews 2:6-7

Many of the old Brothers Grimm fairy tales involved ashes. There were ashes scattered so the heroine can find her way through the dark forest. There were ashes in which the virtuous girl is forced to sleep. Caregivers sometimes feel like Cinderella among the ashes. Often, their works of mercy are unrecognized, seemingly insignificant. But from the dust of the earth God created man in His own image, to love and to be loved. In the end, as Saint John of the Cross said, we will be judged on love.

August 23

Memorabilia

"So faith, hope, love remain, these three; but the greatest of these is love."

— 1 Corinthians 13:13

We are sorting through mementos of my parents' life. They include a World War II Nazi dagger, a collection of Turkish copper pots, a fragment of the Berlin Wall, original paintings, books. How can I part with any of these items that were so precious to my mom and dad? Must I preserve everything in order to honor them properly? But, the memories I hold in my heart are even more precious. I realize that the most valuable thing I can do for them is to pray for them. My love for them reaches beyond the grave.

August 24

Seeing as Jesus Sees

"Faith does not merely gaze at Jesus, but sees things as Jesus himself sees them, with his own eyes: it is a participation in his way of seeing."

— Pope Francis, *Lumen Fidei*

When we see with Christ's eyes, we see that God is not only YHWH (Yahweh), but a loving Father. Perhaps we fear Him a little. After all, God put Abraham to the test, asking him to kill his only son. When Isaac pointed out to his father that they had the wood and the fire, but not the sheep, Abraham told Isaac, "God himself will provide the lamb for a burnt offering" (Gn 22:8, NRSVCE). And Abraham was right. God gives us His only Son, who willingly offered himself for our sake. This is a loving Father. When He asks a sacrifice of us, He provides everything we need to accomplish it.

August 25

A Deep Inner Quiet

"I have calmed and quieted my soul,

like a weaned child with its mother."

— Psalm 131:2, NRSVCE

When we care for someone who cannot speak, we begin to appreciate a special kind of silence. Not the silence that is merely a pause between two speakers, or between thoughts, or an awkward silence that is anxiously waiting to be filled. There is a deeper, more peaceful silence, akin to the stillness of a darkened church when no one is around. It is a church lit only by the sanctuary lamp. This quiet is a peaceful waiting on God, knowing He is upholding us, knowing He is there even when we can't see Him. We feel that inner quiet of a soul resting in God.

AUGUST 26

Speaking Plainly

"His disciples said, 'Now you are talking plainly, and not in any figure of speech. Now we realize that you know everything.'"

— John 16:29

You can just hear them, these poor fishermen, struggling to keep up with the veiled meaning of the parables, with the incisive teaching of the Master. *Now* you're talking plainly! *Now* we know that you are God! Then, Jesus sadly tells them that they will not remain true, especially when the big trouble comes. Just like the disciples, we waver too. When trouble comes, when things aren't going as planned, when God isn't speaking clearly to us, we begin to doubt that God is God. And yet, He reassures us. Take courage!

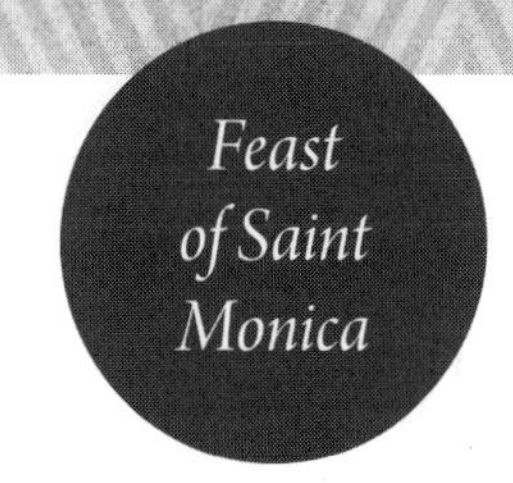

August 27

Perseverance

"And because she loved more than the others, and loving wept, and weeping sought, and seeking persevered, so did she merit to be the first of them all to find Thee, to see Thee, to speak with Thee."

— Saint Augustine, *Confessions*

Isn't it comforting to know that, as Saint Paul tells the Hebrews, we are surrounded by a great cloud of witnesses? Saint Monica is a friend in heaven. She is someone we can call on especially when we feel as though we might not have the strength to persevere. She persevered in prayer and tears for seventeen years, imploring God that her wayward son, Augustine, would become a believer. When we feel burned out, a little despairing, or just plain tired, we can turn to Saint Monica. She never gave up hope. Her tears became a blessing.

August 28

Remember the Promise

"Christ strode through the gate of our final loneliness. . . . [I]n his Passion he went down into the abyss of our abandonment. Where no voice can reach us any longer, there is he."

— Cardinal Joseph Ratzinger, *Introduction to Christianity*

My mom and I are sitting in Dr. Lillian's apartment, admiring her paintings and her view of the forest. She asks me where my mom lives. I tell her it's the twenty-four hour nursing unit several floors below the independent living apartments. Lillian sighs, "That's our biggest fear; that we will fall and end up there." In her case, she explains, it would be even worse, since she has no living relatives who would visit her.

Instead of living in fear, what if we remember the promise? The promise of a future on God's mountain, the snowy majestic peaks high above the clouds, above all tragedy and suffering. All of the loved ones who have passed away, and all the ones we will meet there, will be together with us forever.

August 29

Break Free!

"Prepare the way of the Lord."

— Isaiah 40:3

John the Baptist was beheaded because he had proclaimed the truth. Because Herod's wife could not bear hearing the truth, she told her daughter to demand John's head on a platter. See how evil engenders more evil? The daughter became embroiled in their wickedness. Follow John the Baptist and break the chain of lies that imprison us. By living in the truth, we will be free to love.

August 30

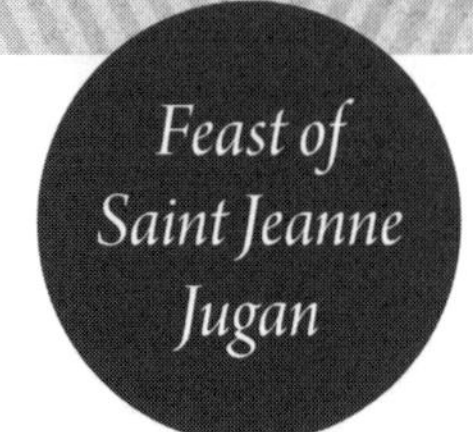

Accompanying Christ

"Love God very much, so that you can look after the aged well, for it is Jesus whom you care for in them."

— Saint Jeanne Jugan

The Little Sisters of the Poor, following the example set by their founder, Saint Jeanne Jugan, care for the elderly as Christ himself would, accompanying them with reverence until God calls them home. What a beautiful mission! All the sisters are eager to be with the dying — even if the call comes during the wee hours of the morning. They will stay with the dying person until the final moment, singing "Salve Regina." Nobody will ever die afraid or alone. The joy of these sisters echoes the example of Jeanne Jugan who lived, as one of her contemporaries said, in the presence of God.

AUGUST 31

Image of God

"Each human being, however wretched or exalted he or she may be, however sick or suffering, however good-for-nothing or important, whether born or unborn, whether incurably ill or radiant with health — each one bears God's breath in himself or herself, each one is God's image."

— *Day to Day with Pope Benedict XVI*

Each day you caregivers live out the two great commandments: love God and love your neighbor. You tend to the basic needs of your loved ones with such delicate charity and attention. Not only do you see God's image in them, but they see God's image in you. It doesn't matter if they are believers, or grateful, or even good.

When the Pharisees accused Jesus of dining with prostitutes and tax collectors, the scum of the Jewish society, He roundly rebuked them: "Go and learn the meaning of the words, 'I desire mercy, not sacrifice'" (Mt 9:13). And we are called to be like Him.

SEPTEMBER 1

Daily Miracle

"The offering to be changed into His Flesh is the most fragile wafer of unleavened bread, light as the petal of a rose. . . . It is this that Christ chooses for His supreme miracle of love."

— Caryll Houselander, *The Passion of the Infant Christ*

Naaman was insulted when the prophet Elisha told him to wash seven times in the Jordan to be cured of his leprosy. There are better rivers in many other places! I have to come to this backwater country to wash in this inferior river? No fanfare, no celebrity doctor, no appearance on *Oprah*? We might think, as Naaman did, that true miracles require lots of drama and plenty of hoopla. Yet what is (seemingly) less dramatic than the miracle of Christ present in the small, white host? The almighty power of God is concentrated in this one particle of bread?

SEPTEMBER 2

Tears of Love

"Bringing an alabaster flask of ointment, she stood behind him at his feet weeping and began to bathe his feet with her tears. Then she wiped them with her hair, kissed them, and anointed them with the ointment."

— Luke 7:37-38

And Jesus tells us that the sins of the woman in the incident referenced above were forgiven because she loved greatly. Caregivers, you also show this great love. The many small details: soothing ointment, a dry towel, holy tears. These amount to great love.

September 3

Fire

"In my sighing a fire blazes up . . .
LORD, let me know my end, the number of my days,
that I may learn how frail I am!"

— Psalm 39:4-5

I am staying at my mom's house when I wake suddenly in the middle of the night. I hear the automated message: "Power failure; please connect power source." I look outside and see the horizon glowing red. I think: nuclear holocaust! Then I open the back door, the door that opens out to the mountains, the dry brush, the desert sage. And I smell the fire. I hunt down flashlights as the fire grows bigger, closer. I pack a bag for my mom, gathering some of her original paintings — the most valuable items (to me) in the house. Eventually, the police show up to evacuate the entire neighborhood.

Fire is all-consuming. Like the Spirit, it blows where it wills. There is a lesson in this: I should remember how frail we creatures are, and how much we depend on the Lord.

SEPTEMBER 4

Compare and Despair

"But, as for me, my feet had almost stumbled;

My steps had nearly slipped,

Because I was envious of the arrogant

When I saw the prosperity of the wicked."

— Psalm 73:2-3

A priest I know sometimes quips, "Compare and despair!" When we start to compare ourselves to someone else, we quickly become discouraged. Why am I such a failure? Or, we become envious. Why is *my* life so difficult?

Comparing leads to discouragement, bitterness, and even despair. Better to keep our eyes fixed on the Lord and trust that He will guide us. He alone is our "stronghold in times of trouble" (Ps 9:10). He will never forsake us.

SEPTEMBER 5

The Path

"In my personal experience with God I cannot do without the path. I would say that one encounters God walking, moving, seeking Him and allowing oneself to be sought by Him. They are two paths that meet. On one hand, there is our path that seeks Him, driven by that instinct that flows from the heart; and after, when we have encountered each other, we realize that He was the one who had been searching for us from the start."

— Cardinal Jorge Mario Bergoglio, *On Heaven and Earth*

I follow the path that runs along the flume, under the aspens and beneath the high desert sky. I have a feeling of exhilaration whenever I run here. It seems like earth meeting sky, where I can reach up to touch heaven. Still, God is always just out of reach. He's in the shaking of the aspen leaves, dawn's glow etching an outline of the mountain. He whispers something I can't quite hear, because my heart isn't empty enough of my worldly desires. I have to be empty and sun bleached like the dry desert driftwood, like the worn path under my feet, or like my mom's pale blue eyes: searching the mountain, searching for her love to call her.

September 6

Sacrifice

"Only by sheltering others do we ourselves receive shelter; only by caring for others will we ourselves find someone to care for us."

— Cardinal Joseph Ratzinger, *Co-Workers of the Truth*

A professor from MIT has written a book warning us about robots that will soon be able to take on all the jobs people don't like. Caregiving, for example. She is an outlier, a voice crying in the wilderness, saying, "This is not a good idea." In 1920, Karel Capek wrote a play about robots (he coined the term) being able to liberate man from Adam's curse: toil. Of course, in his play there was an inevitable holocaust. Without sacrifice, there is no love.

September 7

Time and Presence

"Do not underestimate the value of the time you spend with someone who is suffering. You are afraid because you can't solve the person's problems. Of course you can't. So don't pressure yourself. Give your time. Stay with the person, and be consistent about it. In human things time and presence are the media of love."

— John Janaro, *Never Give Up*

The staff speak respectfully of those who visit daily. Yasmin stops by every morning on her way to work, and there was that one fellow who used to come every day after work and stayed until midnight! They speak of the man in hushed tones. The judge brings his mom a BLT and sits with her during his lunch hour, and Rebecca drives five hours each way to stay with her mom on the weekends. These are small acts, perhaps somewhat insignificant when considered individually. But, over time, they are heroic and speak volumes about love.

Feast of the Birth of Mary

September 8

Master of the Impossible

"Who is this that comes forth like the dawn,

as beautiful as the moon, as resplendent as the sun,

as awe-inspiring as bannered troops?"

— Song of Songs 6:10, NAB

According to tradition, Joachim and Anne were a devout but barren couple whose offering in the Temple was spurned because they had no children. They prayed to God and promised to consecrate their child to His service. An angel appeared and promised that their prayers would be fulfilled. As with Isaac's birth to elderly Sarah, Samuel's birth to the sorrowing Hannah, and John the Baptist's birth to the childless Elizabeth, God revealed His mysterious providence and saving power when things were looking impossible. As Luke's Gospel reminds us, "Nothing will be impossible for God" (1:37).

September 9

Angels Will Support You

"For he commands his angels . . .

to guard you wherever you go.

With their hands they shall support you,

lest you strike your foot against a stone."

— Psalm 91:11-12

One day, as the prophet Habbakuk was cooking his midday meal, an angel suddenly appeared and told him to take dinner to Daniel in the lion's den, in Babylon. Habbakuk protested that he had never seen Babylon nor the lion's den! So the angel picked him up by his hair and, with the speed of the wind, transported him and the dinner to the lion's den. Daniel praised God: "You have not forsaken those who love you" (Dn 14:38).

How truly surprising God is: He could have provided Daniel with a meal any other way. But, He whisked a fellow prophet, a friend who understood, through the air. He shows us that we are meant to be a part of a community. We are not meant to eat alone. And, sometimes, if we trust enough, He can carry us on the wind.

September 10

No Longer Strangers

"By communicating his Spirit, Christ mystically constitutes as his body those brothers of his who are called together from every nation."

— *Catechism of the Catholic Church*, 788

Majid is from Sierra Leone, Eleni is from Ethiopia, Blanca from Mexico. This place is like the United Nations in multicolored scrubs! And all are committed to healing, to creating a space of hospitality and comfort. In the end, the voice that sounds like a multitude or like rushing water (see Rv 14:2) will call the suffering ones. It will call the martyred ones, and the persecuted ones, and all those who have been washed in the ocean of His mercy to the wedding feast of the Lamb.

September 11

The Battle Is the Lord's

"Where are the Hittites? Why does no one find it remarkable that in most world cities today there are Jews but not one single Hittite, even though the Hittites had a great flourishing civilization while the Jews were a weak and obscure people?"

— Walker Percy, *The Message in the Bottle*

Over and over again in Scripture we see that God chooses the weak, the seemingly inconsequential, to do His great works. David versus Goliath. Gideon's army was reduced from tens of thousands to a mere 300 men. When Joshua leads his army in the siege against Jericho, God tells them to march around the city blowing their horns. We need to have this message drilled into our hearts because we creatures always try to take all the credit. God wants us to know that the battle is the Lord's.

SEPTEMBER 12

Boomerang Peace

"As you enter a house, wish it peace. If the house is worthy, let your peace come upon it; if not, let your peace return to you."

— Matthew 10:12-13

When I enter the nursing home, I say: "Hello, how are you? It's a beautiful day!" And everyone — the residents and staff alike — greets me back with remarkable good cheer. The always smiling World War II vet, with his U.S. Marine Corps baseball cap, wheezes, "Howdy, Ma'am!" The janitor with his eyes twinkling, blesses me: "Have a blessed day." I feel God's peace resting on this place and coming back to me, too.

SEPTEMBER 13

The Last Will Be First

"Go out quickly into the streets and alleys of the town and bring in here the poor and the crippled, the blind and the lame."

— Luke 14:21

In Flannery O'Connor's short story *Revelation*, the main character is a hardworking, rather Pharisaical (in the same way I often am), Southern farm woman who considers herself a good Christian. She is thankful she isn't like other people. Mrs. Turpin has a vision while tending the hogs. She sees "a vast horde of souls all rumbling toward heaven." They are white-trash, the freaks and lunatics, singing off-key, jumping and clapping, leading the way to paradise, while dignified people like herself bring up the rear.

Compared to the almighty God, creator of heaven and earth, we are all on the level of the pig farmer. Not one of us is better than the other, and we are all equally dependent on His grace.

SEPTEMBER 14

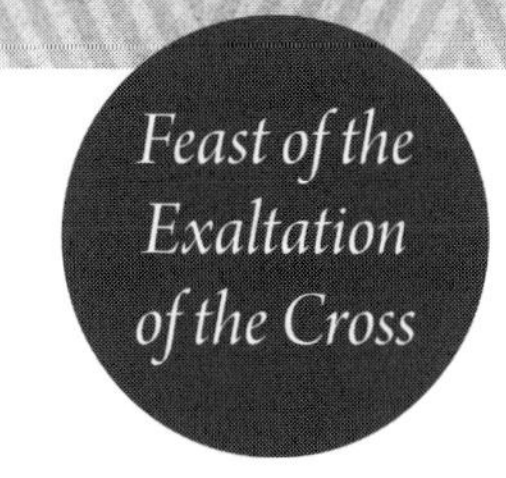

Lifted Up

"And just as Moses lifted up the serpent in the desert, so must the Son of Man be lifted up, so that everyone who believes in him might have eternal life."

— John 3:14

In the desert, the Israelites grumbled and complained, "We are disgusted with this wretched food!" This food was, in fact, the miraculous manna that God blessed them with every single day. So, God punished them by sending venomous snakes among them. When the people repented, God told Moses to put a bronze serpent on a pole. Anyone who looked upon it would recover (see Nm 21:4-9).

Jesus was lifted up on the cross, on which we find our salvation. Being lifted up sometimes does not look beautiful in the moment. But after the Cross, there is the Resurrection.

SEPTEMBER 15

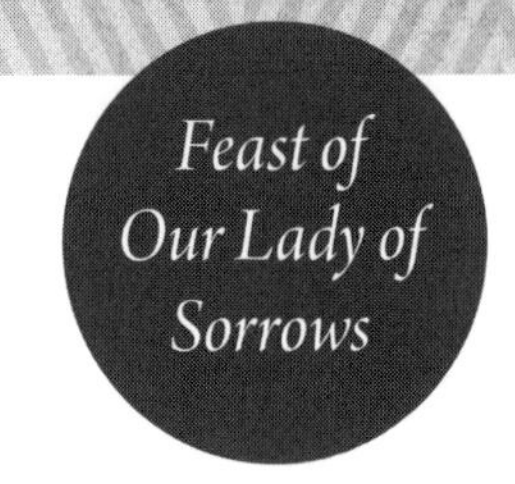

The Dawn

"Who can be a better star of hope for us than she, the dawn that announced the day of salvation?"

— Pope Benedict, *Angelus*, December 8, 2007

Sometimes, Courtney's seizures last so long that her mom fears she will not recover. There is no greater pain than watching helplessly while your child suffers. In the midst of fear and trembling, as your heart is stricken, you may briefly fear that God has forsaken you. But as my dad used to say, "It's always darkest before the dawn."

Our Blessed Mother, the woman of Seven Sorrows, also watched her innocent son suffer. She can comfort us during the worst trials. She is the cause of our joy, the morning star. Mary brings the dawn, shining with new hope. She shows us the grace we need in the midst of the darkest darkness.

September 16

Everyone Has Something to Give

"People whose demand on others is simple and uncomplicated add to the life of the world."

— Caryll Houselander, *The Passion of the Infant Christ*

My mom and all those in nursing homes or at home in their sickbeds have very simple and uncomplicated demands. They wish to be fed, to be clean and warm, to be comfortable. Most of all, they love visitors. My mom greets every one she sees with an enthusiastic wave and smile. She loves equally the gardener, the housekeeper who empties the trash, the doctors, and the nurses. She is adding to the inner life of the world.

September 17

God's Bounty

"The world is charged with the grandeur of God."

— Gerard Manley Hopkins, *God's Grandeur*

Around noontime, the apostle Peter went up to the terrace on the roof to pray. We imagine Peter, sleepy from hunger, his eyes closed in prayer. As the sun beat down hot upon the terrace, he fell into a trance. Not a single cloud marred the perfect sapphire sky. Suddenly, through a rent in the endless blue, a shimmering sheet with all kinds of animals, birds, and reptiles floated down. A voice told Peter to slaughter and eat. Though he objected, the voice commanded him: "What God has made clean, you are not to call profane" (Acts 10:15). Through every creature, every flower, every tree top and mountain, every blue sky, and even every moment, God gives of himself. He is bountiful.

September 18

The Dying of Jesus

"But we hold this treasure in earthen vessels, that the surpassing power may be of God and not from us. We are afflicted in every way, but not constrained; perplexed, but not driven to despair; persecuted, but not abandoned; struck down, but not destroyed; always carrying about in the body the dying of Jesus, so that the life of Jesus may also be manifested in our body."

— 2 Corinthians 4:7-10

Mr. A. is perplexed through Alzheimer's. My mom was struck down by a stroke. Lillian is alone in Gethsemane, with no living relatives. Irene carries Jesus' cross, a burden that is so heavy, she cannot rise from her hospital bed. Mrs. X. is scourged every day by her bitter memories. Arne is nailed to the cross of caring for his wife with MS. All who suffer being changed and dressed and fed every day suffer the humiliation of the crowning of thorns. All are carrying the dying of Jesus. Not because there was anything lacking in Jesus, but because we need to see the life of Christ manifested in us, in our bodies.

SEPTEMBER 19

The God of Perpetual Surprises

"Religious man is a wayfarer; he must be ready to let himself be led, to come out of himself and to find the God of perpetual surprises."

— Pope Francis, *Lumen Fidei*

Just catching a glimpse of the huge Irish wolfhound makes everyone at the nursing home laugh. "Shock and awe," explains Blackie's owner. He visits nursing homes and children's hospitals, bringing them the joy and surprise of a lovable furry giant. God surprises us, too, when He answers our prayers in an unexpected way. Did Daniel expect lunch to be served via an angel and a fellow prophet in the lion's den? Did Martha and Mary expect their brother to come stumbing out of the grave, wrapped in putrid burial cloths? Watch for the surprise, wait for it.

SEPTEMBER 20

Living Every Nasty Moment

"Some days I feel as if I want to die, but I can't. I have to live every nasty moment. Everything hurts. Everything is degrading. My consciousness is dominated by various physical dysfunctions, and I mark time."

— John Janaro, *Never Give Up*

When I try to put myself in my mom's place, or in Irene's, or in Mr. D.'s, who isn't even aware that he lives here, I think, "Just shoot me now!" But then I remember that even when everything seems most hopeless, even when the sufferer himself prays for death (like Tobit and Sarah who prayed that God would end their lives) God has a plan for each one of us. He has counted every hair on our heads. And we trust that this present suffering will be completely subsumed by the future joy.

But it's not just about waiting and hanging on by the skin of our teeth until this present life is over. God wants to transform even the present moment. Let us pray for transformation, even the nasty moments.

September 21

Loving Your Enemy

"And so I discovered that it is not on our forgiveness any more than on our goodness that the world's healing hinges, but on His. When He tells us to love our enemies, He gives, along with the command, the love itself."

— Corrie Ten Boom, *The Hiding Place*

When Jesus teaches us how to pray, He also tells us that we must forgive those who have hurt us. He says that if you do not forgive others, neither will your Father forgive your transgressions (see Mt 6:15). This is huge! It is as important as the Ten Commandments! Yet, how often do we remain locked in our anger, resentment, and bitterness about past hurts? The first step is to ask Jesus to help you. You can't change the past, or even your feelings, but you can ask Christ to help you forgive.

SEPTEMBER 22

Worthy Are Tested

"Accept whatever happens to you;

in periods of humiliation be patient.

For in fire gold is tested,

and the chosen in the crucible of humiliation."

— Ben Sira (Sirach) 2:4-5

See, both you and the one for whom you care are golden. God tests the worthy. It takes humility and patience to be a caregiver and to accept caregiving.

September 23

Paradise

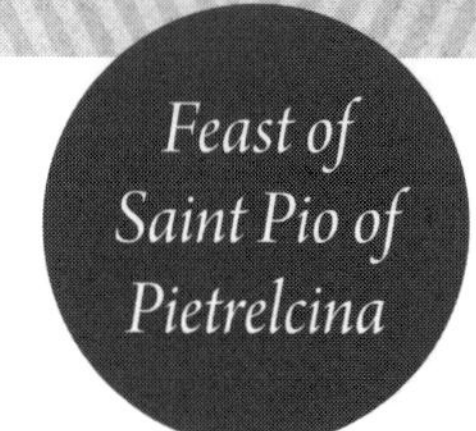

"Where there is no obedience, there is no virtue; where there is no virtue, there is no goodness, no love; and where there is no love there is no God: without God we do not go to Paradise."

— Padre Pio, *Quotable Saints*

We can count on Padre Pio, especially when we find ourselves worrying about whether we can get everything done (wanting to be in two places at once) and wishing we could cure our sick loved ones. Padre Pio bore the stigmata (the wounds of Christ) and was known to bilocate. Many were healed through his intercession. One time, he was at home in San Giovanni Rotondo in a trance. At the same moment, it turns out, he was giving absolution to a dying man in another city. An American World War II bombardier pilot was saved over the Pacific Ocean when his parachute failed to open. He was carried to the ground by someone he only later recognized as Padre Pio. His mother had entrusted him to the saint.

Padre Pio promised that he would stand at the threshold of paradise until all his spiritual children entered. Let us pray that we are accepted as one of his spiritual children.

September 24

A Future Filled with Hope

"The more experience I have with the older sisters, the more I realize how few of us hope simply to survive. We want to retain our ability to reason, to remember, to express our thoughts, to read a new novel or the newspaper. . . . We want to live in communities with people we love and people who love us. In short, we want to have what Sister Genevieve has — including, odd as it might sound for a woman who is now ninety years old, a future filled with hope."

— David Snowdon, *Aging with Grace*

Her husband has died and now, with her memory faltering and nobody to care for her, she finds herself living at the nursing home in the Alzheimer's unit. She's holding a dog-eared twelve-year-old guidebook to Rome, smiling. We ask, "Are you planning a trip?" She answers delightedly, "Yes!" She thinks maybe this year, with her husband.

SEPTEMBER 25

Bruised Reed

"A bruised reed he will not break,

a smoldering wick he will not quench."

— Matthew 12:20

She is the bruised reed — so delicate, helpless, and trusting. I manage to get us in front of the big Westminster chiming clock at precisely the right moment. As the chimes begin, her blue eyes go wide. She is a child again. Perhaps it reminds her of her own Westminster chiming clock. I watch her listening attentively. God loves the bruised reed, and allows the flame to smolder until it's time.

SEPTEMBER 26

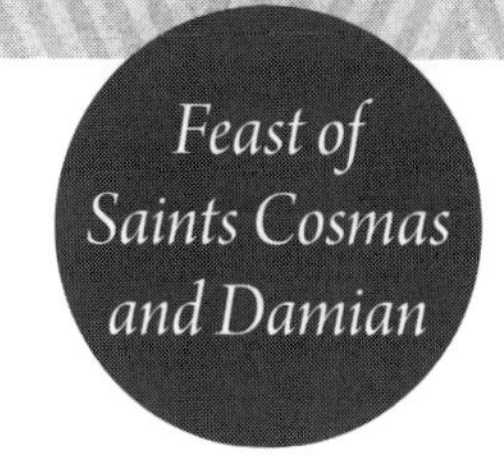

Hymn of Praise

"Suffering — without ceasing to be suffering — becomes, despite everything, a hymn of praise"

— Pope Benedict XVI, *Spe Salvi*

In a seaport town on the Gulf of Iskenderun, on the edge of the brilliant blue of the Mediterranean Sea, twin brothers Cosmas and Damian, both physicians, practiced medicine. They healed the sick for free, earning them the nickname "the silverless." They never recanted under torture for their faith — despite being hung, stoned, shot with arrows, and finally beheaded. In Fra Angelico's painting, the two martyrs are pictured blindfolded, kneeling, blood spurting heavenward, their severed heads lying on the ground.

Let us pray for perseverance in suffering, with the heavenly assistance of these two physician saints.

SEPTEMBER 28

God at the Door

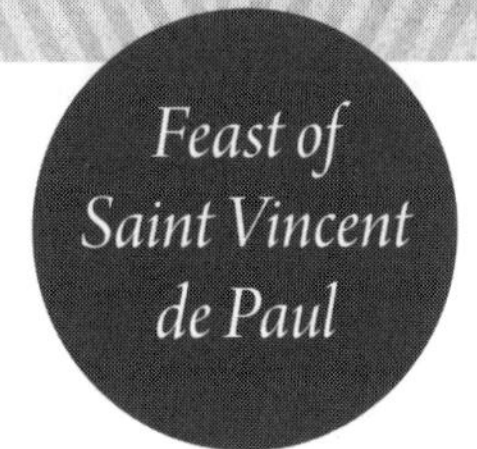

"If a needy person requires medicine or other help during prayer time, do whatever has to be done with peace of mind. . . . When you leave prayer to serve some poor person, remember that this very service is performed for God."

— Saint Vincent de Paul, *Epistle 2546*

Saint Vincent de Paul spent the first ten years of his priesthood rather indifferently, hoping to land a well-paying position in the Church. Under the direction of several holy priests, he experienced a gradual conversion both to his vocation and to love for the poor. He took care of galley slaves, victims of war, the sick, abandoned children, and impoverished country people.

He even made time to found the Congregation of the Missions — known as the Vincentians, who had a particular concern for the rural poor. He founded, with Saint Louise de Marillac, the Daughters of Charity. The scope of his charitable works was staggering, but he did it with a simplicity that flowed from faith. "Nothing pleases me except in Jesus Christ," he once said.

St. Vincent embodied Jesus' admonition: "Whatever you did for one of these least brothers of mine, you did for me" (Mt 25:40).

September 29

The Angels' Mission

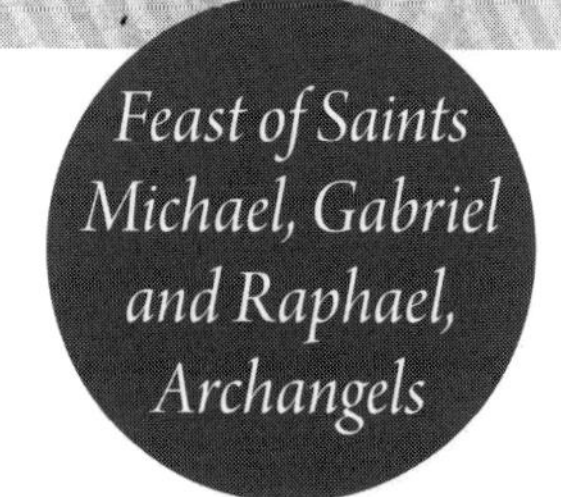

"Love grants prophecy, miracles. It is an abyss of illumination, a fountain of fire, bubbling up to inflame the thirsty soul. It is the condition of angels, and the progress of eternity."

— John Climacus, *The Ladder of Divine Ascent*

Saint Michael wields the sword, protecting us against prowling demons. Gabriel seems the gentle messenger. (I love Lorenzo Lotto's painting of the Annunciation, with a sweetly surprised Mary, a scared cat, and the beautiful angel Gabriel himself looking awed as he brings the news.) But my favorite archangel is Raphael, who is a master of disguise as well as being a brilliant matchmaker. He cures Tobit of his blindness and drives the demon Asmodeus out of Sarah. We should pray today to the archangels for protection and healing.

September 30

Feast of Saint Jerome

Reward for Your Labor

"It was many years ago when, for the sake of the kingdom of heaven, I had cut myself off from my home, my parents, my sister, my kinsmen, and — what was even more difficult — from an accustomed habit of good living. I was going to Jerusalem to be a soldier of Christ."

— Saint Jerome, *Letters of St. Jerome*

Saint Jerome was known for having a very difficult temperament. He was quarrelsome, argumentative, and struggled throughout his life with his temper. Yet, despite this, he became a saint. His inability to get along with people might even be part of the reason he left his home to live as a hermit in the Holy Land. And it is there that he accomplished his greatest work — translating the Scriptures from Hebrew into Latin. Though he struggled his whole life with his own boiling moods, he nonetheless achieved sanctity through his heroic virtue. Isn't it comforting to know that God uses even the difficult or troublesome aspects of our human nature to accomplish His work?

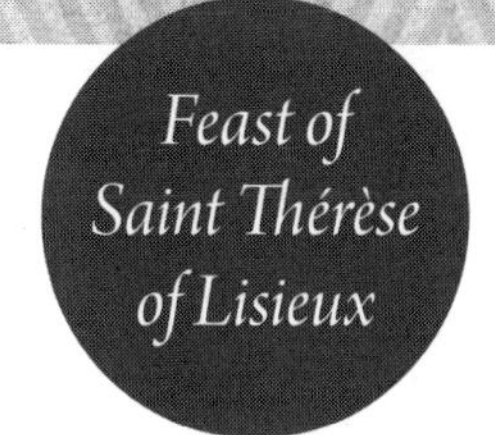

October 1

The Little Way

"I am a very little soul who can offer very little things to God."

— Saint Thérèse of Lisieux, *The Story of a Soul*

Saint Thérèse used to take care of a demanding, elderly nun, gently helping her walk to the dining room. All the while, she listened to the old woman's complaints: "You're walking too fast; I shall fall! I knew you were too young to look after me!" But, Saint Thérèse gave the old woman her "nicest smile" and tenderly looked after her. One cold and dark winter evening, Thérèse heard an orchestra and, for a moment, somewhat wistfully imagined a party of fashionably dressed young women at a richly decorated home. Then Thérèse looked at the poor invalid with all her complaints and was moved by the contrast. In that moment, she realized that she would not exchange ten minutes with the poor invalid for a thousand years of such parties. She saw in that moment what is most pleasing to God.

October 2

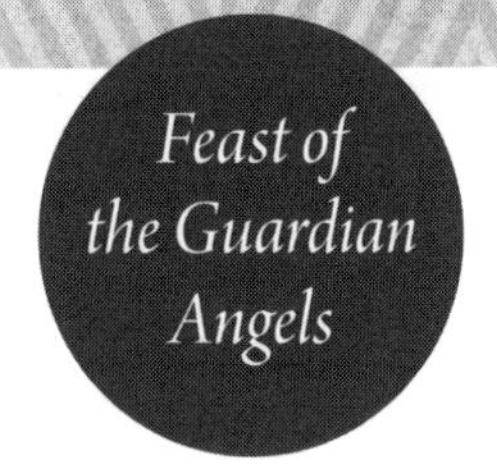

Standing Guard

"How great the dignity of the soul, since each one has from his birth an angel commissioned to guard it."

— Saint Jerome

Jacob dreamed of a stairway going all the way to heaven, with angels ascending and descending. And God told him, "I am with you and will protect you wherever you go" (Gn 28:15). Before her stroke, I would help my mom up and down the few stairs into her house. I would hold the walker steady and she would grip the railing until she was back on firm ground. Those two steps were treacherous, and I was so relieved and grateful to be there to give her assistance. When I wasn't there to help, I entrusted her to the guardian angels, who are good with stairs.

October 3

The Unexpected Christ

"God is always first and makes the first move. ... We read it in the Prophets. God is encountered walking, along the path. ... God is always a surprise, so you never know where and how you will find him. You are not setting the time and place of the encounter with him. You must, therefore, discern the encounter."

— Pope Francis, "A Big Heart Open to God," interview with Anthony Spadaro, S.J., *America Magazine*, September 30, 2013

My friend Robin's dad was stuck in the rehab facility. He called his daughter daily, sometimes two, three times a day. "I am so cold!" he exclaimed. "This place is freezing!" Why don't you put on a sweater, Dad?" suggested Robin. "That won't work! It's just so cold here. I've never been so cold in my life!" "Can you ask them to turn down the air conditioning in your room?" Her dad groaned. "My hands are like blocks of ice!" Robin switched tactics, and tried empathic listening instead. "Gosh, Dad, that's just terrible!" "What!?" her dad shouts, "What are you saying? Now you're scaring me!"

October 4

Tenderness

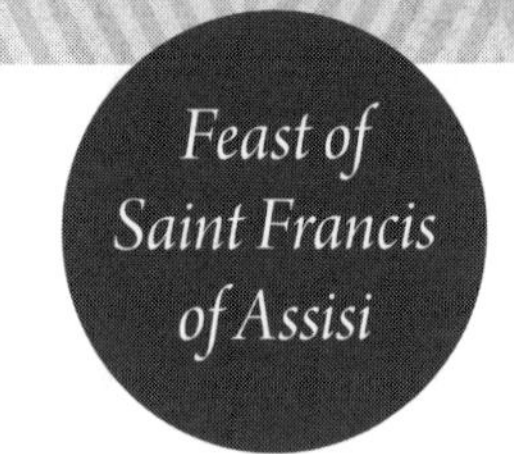

"There are people who leave behind, so to speak, a surplus of love, of perseverance in suffering, of honor and truth that captures others and sustains them."

— Pope Benedict XVI, *Images of Hope*

The saints are our brothers and sisters in heaven who, going before us, show us how to love better, how to persevere in hope despite suffering. Saint Francis, one of the most beloved of saints, captures our hearts and imagination. When his father threatened to disinherit him, Francis did one better. He renounced his inheritance and then stripped off his clothes and returned those as well.

His effusive love for all creatures extended even to wild animals. His tender love for the infant Jesus manifested itself in the creation of the first crèche. In giving us this manager scene, Francis showed us a face of God that is so near to us, so gentle and helpless. It has inspired us to share this tender love with the most vulnerable.

October 5

God's Hidden Face

"This is God's way with us, to hide and reveal himself at the same time; to show His desire for man's love, making himself accessible, even ordinary, that He may come close, yet at the same time playing a game of hide and seek, saying 'Seek and you shall find.'"

— Caryll Houselander, *The Passion of the Infant Christ*

Scripture tells us that Moses spoke to God "face to face" — intimately, as to a friend. Yet, he never actually saw the face of God. When Moses asked to see His glory, God told him that He would pass by and allow Moses to see His back, because no man sees God's face and lives. This is the gentleness of God's approach. He doesn't reveal himself all at once because it would kill us. With delicate charity, He shows us His back, as He is passing by. We get a sense, an intimation. What if that was God? What if that kind janitor who wished me a mysterious blessing was God passing by?

October 6

God Needs You

"That you need God more than anything, you know at all times in your heart. But don't you know also that God needs you — in the fullness of his eternity, you?"

— Martin Buber, *I and Thou*

One tear shed by the infant Christ could have been sufficient to save the entire world. But, God chose to allow His only Son to suffer the indignities of life, the agony of His Passion, and cruel death on the Cross. And God did not need the young teenage girl from the backwater town, but He chose her out of all eternity to be the mother of His Son. He lifts up the lowly and scatters the proud-hearted.

Little hunchback Nellie laboriously trundles her walker over the pathway to greet us: "It makes me so happy," she breathes, "to see your mom outside on a beautiful day like today." You may think you have nothing to offer, but God chooses to need you.

October 7

Victory Rosary

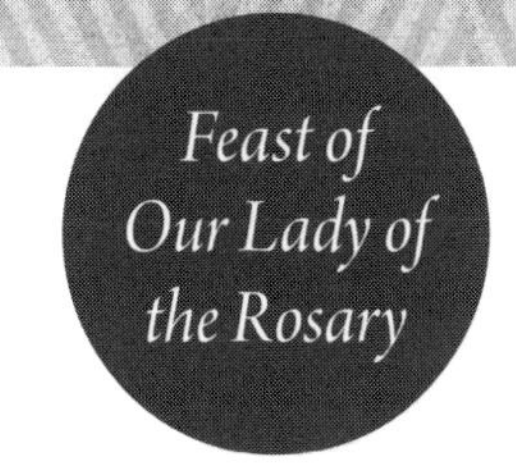

"To pray the Rosary is to hand over our burdens to the merciful hearts of Christ and his Mother."

— Saint John Paul II, *Apostolic Letter on the Rosary*

On this date in 1571, the powerful fleet of the Ottoman Empire was decisively defeated by the Holy League, at the great sea battle of Lepanto. After fasting for three days, Don John of Austria, leading the makeshift Christian fleet at the behest of Pope Pius V, sailed for Lepanto. At the same time, the pope asked all the people of Rome to pray the Rosary. As the Turkish ships advanced, John knelt down to pray. At this very moment, the wind changed to favor the Christian ships. In the painting by Paolo Veronese, we see a crush of ships entangled beneath the clouds of heaven, lightning and flaming arrows pouring down. Above the clouds, we see saints and angels, kneeling and pleading before Our Lady. Pope Pius declared the date of the battle the feast of the Most Holy Rosary. To this day, historians are not sure why the outnumbered Christian fleet, fighting on Turkish waters, got the best of the more powerful Ottoman fleet.

Let us remember that Our Lady watches over each one of us even though our battles may be small. We can ask her to help us.

October 8

Never Abandoned

"Say to [your wife], 'Our time here is brief and fleeting, but if we are pleasing to God, we can exchange this life for the Kingdom to come. Then we will be perfectly one both with Christ and each other, and our pleasure will know no bounds.'"

— Saint John Chrysostom, *Homily on Ephesians*

My parents (married more than sixty years) did almost everything together, especially once my dad retired from the military. It was grocery shopping on Wednesday, Red Lobster on Friday, Sunday Mass followed by brunch at Heidi's Pies or the Peppermill. Except for Saturdays, when my dad went to the Y to play handball and out for a burger with his buddies, they were inseparable. So, my mom felt abandoned, deeply stricken, when her best friend and constant companion was called home.

But, we are never really alone or abandoned. We are loved by God every moment of our existence. Those of you who care for loved ones in many physical ways can remind them each day that they are loved by God. They are never abandoned.

October 9

We Are All Responsible

"For know, dear ones, that every one of us is undoubtedly responsible for all men and everything on earth, not merely through the general sinfulness of creation, but each one personally for all mankind and every individual man."

— Fyodor Dostoyevsky, *The Brothers Karamazov*

Jesus assures us that God will quickly answer those who call out to Him, day and night, seeking justice. "But when the Son of Man comes, will he find faith on earth?" (Lk 18:8). On that fateful day, the day when His justice flashes like lightning from the east to the west, the Lord will ask us: "Why didn't you feed me when I was hungry? Why didn't you visit me in prison? Why didn't you clothe me when I was naked? Why did you care only about your own home, your own well-being, your own small part of the world?"

We are, each one of us, personally responsible for everyone. And no small act of kindness, no sip of water for those who cry out to God, will be unnoticed.

OCTOBER 10

Don't Try to Solve It All Yourself

"So often in life we ought to slow down and not try to fix everything at once! To travel in patience means these things: it's giving up the presumption of wanting to solve everything. You have to make an effort, but understand that one person cannot do everything."

— Pope Francis, *Conversations with Jorge Bergoglio: His Life in His Own Words*

When we are baptized, we enter into a community. Our faith is not something private, just for me alone. Our faith is believing together. It's the faith of our fathers, the faith of the Church. Each of us is, as Pope Francis says, a link in this chain of love. And so, when we want to fix things, solve the world's problems, or our own, we should realize that we don't have to go it alone. We are part of a community of believers. We can ask for help.

October 11

Lesser and Greater Hopes

"In our many different sufferings and trials we always need the lesser and greater hopes too — a kind visit, the healing of internal and external wounds, a favorable resolution of a crisis."

— Pope Benedict XVI, *Spe Salvi*

Irene wants me to help her make a phone call to follow up on a new job application. She has decided not to go for the job in Barstow, Alaska. She decides to try for something closer to home. Her sister helps her fill out the application, as Irene is confined to bed in a nursing home. Since the stroke affected her eyesight, she asks me to read off the phone number while she dials with her one working arm. We try several times and I am worrying that someone might actually answer the phone. Then the conversation could become awkward. Thankfully, the number is busy is each time, though Irene suspects she might have misdialed. We agree to try another time, perhaps after her nap. Her hopeful perseverance is inspiring.

October 12

The Abyss

"For he afflicts and shows mercy,

Casts down to the depths of Hades,

Brings up from the great abyss."

— Tobit 13:2

"In the beginning . . . the earth was a formless wasteland, and *darkness covered the abyss*" (Gn 1:1-2, NAB). God brings us out of that abyss. Do you sometimes feel, as a caregiver, that you are in an abyss of drudgery and exhaustion? Day after day, the same routine can seem monotonous and unfulfilling, thankless. Yet, God sends His only Son to go down into hell, into the dark abyss. Jesus endures the mockery and derision of those He loves, the agony and death on the Cross, the descent into hell. Is our day really so bad? God sheds His light of love on us, sends His spirit to lift our hearts, gives us the strength to continue.

October 13

Jar of Flour, Jug of Oil

"Let justice descend, you heavens, like dew from above,

like gentle rain let the clouds drop it down.

Let the earth open and salvation bud forth;

let righteousness spring up with them!"

— Isaiah 45:8

Elijah the Tishbite, having prophesied a drought upon the land, seeks out a widow of Zarephath, obeying the Lord's instruction. When he asks for a bit of bread, the widow agreed reluctantly, for this was her last handful of flour. She expected that she and her son would die. Elijah told her that "the jar of flour shall not go empty, nor the jug of oil run dry, until the day when the Lord sends rain upon the earth" (1 Kgs 17:14).

Just like the widow of Zarephath, my mom has little left on earth. So little is needed to sustain her. I trust that God will not let her jug of oil run dry until the day He sends His blessing rain.

October 14

Vision in the Sanctuary

"Meanwhile the people were waiting for Zechariah and were amazed that he stayed so long in the sanctuary. But when he came out, he was unable to speak to them, and they realized that he had seen a vision in the sanctuary."

— Luke 1:21-22

Zechariah could not speak because he didn't believe the words of the angel Gabriel. The demoniac was mute because he was possessed by a demon (see Mt 12:22). Jesus healed the mute man by touching the man's tongue with His own saliva (Mk 7:31-37). This, after He breathed a deep sigh from the depths of His spirit. The speech therapist says my mom is not progressing, even though she was able to say "Wonderful" and sing Happy Birthday. He says we "tricked" her brain into these manifestations of involuntary speech. I dream about us talking again. I have so many questions. Has she perhaps seen a vision in the sanctuary?

October 15

You Go, Girl!

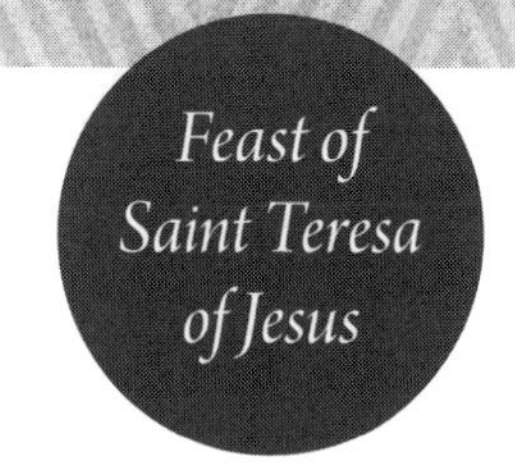

"Within each soul there is a mansion for God."

— Saint Teresa of Jesus, *Interior Castle*

When she was only seven years old, Teresa ran away from home in Avila (dragging her brother with her) and hoping to become a martyr in Africa. Fortunately, they hadn't gone far when they were discovered by her uncle. Saint Teresa is one of three women Doctors of the Church and a reformer of the Carmelite order. She founded convents and monasteries despite persecution from within the Church by those opposed to her efforts to return to the austere roots of the Carmelite way of life. After five hundred years, these convents are still thriving.

Gifted with zeal, piety, sharp business acumen, and a wonderful sense of humor, she wrote many books on prayer and the mystical life. She was often plain-spoken and practical. "God wants your soul to experience heavenly bliss, now and for all eternity," she once said. "Would you like to accept or decline?"

When we feel attacked by the ones who should be on our side, when we encounter trials and setbacks, let's remember how Saint Teresa persevered. We should ask her to intercede for us.

OCTOBER 16

The Bucket List

"I'm starting to consider the fact that I have to leave everything behind. But I take it as something that's normal. I'm not sad. It makes me want to be fair with everyone always, to sign the final flourish."

— Pope Francis, *Conversations with Jorge Bergoglio: His Life in His Own Words*

The Promised Land was probably Number One on Moses' bucket list. He led the grumbling, whining Israelites for forty years through the desert, all the while teaching them, admonishing them, revealing God's word to them. Yet, because of one transgression, God would not permit him to cross the Jordan. Moses died on the mountain overlooking the Promised Land.

Many of us, whether through aging, illness or death, will never complete our bucket lists. This may be a blessing in disguise. God gave Moses something better than the Promised Land: eternal life. This is a reminder that I should worry more about my eternal soul than about fulfilling my every earthly dream.

OCTOBER 17

Become Like Little Children

"Thus it is that many fulfill the condition for entering the Kingdom of Heaven, suffering their desolation with the child's undiluted capacity for suffering but with death robbed of its terror by the child's capacity for perfect trust."

— Caryll Houselander, *The Reed of God*

Mr. D. is sitting in his wheelchair with one shoe off and one shoe on, like in the nursery rhyme. He greets us politely, and my mom acknowledges him with a gracious nod. He tells me he is thinking about living here permanently, but he is still checking it out. "It's a very confusing place," he points out. "I'd better think about it." The nurses call out, "Mr. D., where's your other shoe?"

Jesus tells us that we cannot enter the kingdom of heaven unless we become like little children. Here in the nursing home, so many are like little children — helpless, trusting, dependent on caregivers for every personal need. Here are the childlike — completely dependent on the love of their Father God. They will enter the kingdom of God straightway.

OCTOBER 18

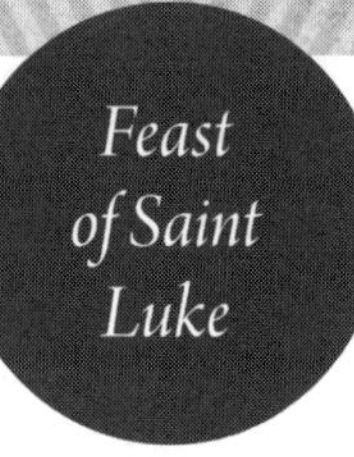

Crown of Righteousness

"Luke, the beloved physician . . . "

— Colossians 4:14

Saint Luke, born a pagan, was from Antioch in ancient Syria, according to an early source. He traveled with Saint Paul on missionary journeys. He composed the third Gospel as well as the Acts of the Apostles. When Saint Paul was imprisoned in Rome before his martyrdom, Paul wrote, "Luke is the only one with me" (2 Tm 4:11).

Because he was a doctor and is the patron saint of physicians, and because he remained with Paul during his final days of imprisonment, he is an appropriate intercessor on behalf of our loved ones. Let's ask him to offer healing blessings during the imprisonment of their illness. Let's pray that they will not be alone or abandoned in their final hours.

October 19

A Future Full of Hope

"The just shall flourish like the palm tree,

Shall grow like a cedar of Lebanon.

Planted in the house of the LORD,

They shall flourish in the courts of our God."

— Psalm 92:13-14

For my mother, this life now is a bitter valley. It is now a life without her beloved husband of six decades. She is without the one she knew from the moment she first saw him. He was a twenty-five-year-old striding in with his boots from the field. No boring desk job for him . . . *This is the one I will marry!* For sixty-four years, she loved him. And yet, as her body grows weaker, she walks strong in spirit toward the one who calls her. They will be reunited in the courts of the Lord.

October 20

Heaven Watching

"So is it, with the Christ-life in each of us and in the world. It is lodged in little ones, in the weakest and puniest, and love and death stand over it face to face."

— Caryll Houselander, *Passion of the Infant Christ*

Archbishop Fulton Sheen once said that when we are well, we are looking forward or else down at our feet. But when we are ill, we are lying in bed looking heavenward. Or, and this is even more likely, heaven is looking down on us! We can imagine all the saints, our own special name saints, as well as our family members in heaven, plus our own special guardian angel, watching out over us when we are sick. It's comforting to think that all of heaven is watching over our dear, sick ones.

October 21

Anguish in the Garden

"Even today that Garden [of Olives] shelters some very ancient olive trees. Perhaps they witnessed what happened beneath their shade that evening, when Christ in prayer was filled with anguish 'and his sweat became like drips of blood falling down upon the ground.'"

— Saint John Paul II, *Ecclesia de Eucharistia*

At least once a day, I hear the ominous sound of the ambulance sirens. I hold my breath as paramedics run in with a stretcher. When we see such anguish, loneliness, physical suffering, and, at times, even blood, we can only place our dear ones in the hands of Jesus. They are hands that were bloodied and pierced by nails, hands that offered himself up as salvation for everyone. Jesus offered His own blood for our redemption, pouring himself out for us.

OCTOBER 22

Mustard-Seed-Sized Faith

"[Faith] is the lifelong companion that makes it possible to perceive, ever anew, the marvels that God works for us."

— Pope Benedict XVI, *Porta Fidei*

When the disciples asked Jesus why they couldn't drive out a demon, Jesus replies: "If you have faith the size of a mustard seed. . . . Nothing will be impossible for you" (Mt 17:20). Like me in so many situations, the disciples *want* to perform a miracle . . . but can't. Even faith the size of a mustard seed can be hard to come by.

The truth is that faith isn't something already out there. We can't roll up to the drive-through window and order a supersized chunk. It's a gift from God, planted in our souls, and we must water the seedling so it can grow.

October 23

Light and Serenity

Feast of Saint John of Capistrano

"By the brightness of their holiness they must bring light and serenity to all who gaze on them. They have been placed here to care for others."

— Saint John of Capistrano, *Mirror of the Clergy*

Caregivers, you bring light and serenity to those for whom you care! My sister-in-law loves to give her ninety-four-year-old mom a spa day. Spa day includes hair trim and blow dry, manicure, massage, make-up, and perfume. Though her mom hasn't spoken for ten years, her eyes light up and she squeezes her daughter's hand in gratitude. Each one of us — despite our limitations and failings — is called to bring light and serenity to others.

October 24

Angels in the Desert

"The angel of the Lord spoke to Philip, 'Get up and head south on the road that goes down from Jerusalem to Gaza, the desert route.'"

— Acts 8:26

How often are the angels speaking to us, though we simply aren't listening? Go to Gaza, take the desert route. An unlikely request! And here Philip meets a most unlikely person, a eunuch reading Isaiah. The eunuch asks Philip to explain the Scripture.

Who are the unlikely characters we might need to meet in the desert? The desert might be the lonely barren trail, or it might be the nursing home where the unloved and forgotten spend their days waiting for someone to bring the love of Jesus Christ to them.

October 25

Mr. and Mrs. Whiner

"And a Christian who constantly complains, fails to be a good Christian: they become Mr. or Mrs. Whiner, no? Because they always complain about everything, right? Silence in endurance, silence in patience. That silence of Jesus: Jesus in His Passion did not speak much, only two or three necessary words. . . . But it is not a sad silence: the silence of bearing the Cross is not a sad silence. It is painful, often very painful, but it is not sad. The heart is at peace."

— Pope Francis, *Homily*, May 7, 2013

The psychiatrist asks my mom if she ever feels depressed. She bursts out laughing. "I guess that's a no," he says wryly. I am dumbfounded. My mom hasn't laughed this hard since the time I pretended I was Danny Kaye in the film *The Court Jester*, dueling the villain while under the spell of the witch. Even better, I know her heart is at peace.

October 26

The Slavery of Selfishness

"The path we follow toward genuine loving leads by way of losing oneself and through all the affliction of an Exodus."

— Cardinal Joseph Ratzinger, *God and Love*

God led the Israelites out of slavery and into the desert. There, they complained and grumbled, "We would rather *die* in Egypt with our fleshpots, than starve out here in the desert!" Pope Benedict XVI says that everyone has to undergo his own Exodus. We have to leave the comfortable — yet isolated — land of the self. And sometimes, we would rather *die* than truly, genuinely, extend ourselves to another. We risk embarrassment and rejection.

Loving means transcending ourselves. It means leaving behind the slavery of our selfishness. Each day brings a new opportunity to love.

October 27

The Gift of Tears

"Our tears can lead us to the heart of Jesus who wept for our world."

— *Mornings with Henri Nouwen*

One of the best nurses is on duty today — after pulling several all-nighters. His eyes are bloodshot, yet he struggles to give a cheerful greeting. Sometimes, caregivers can feel stretched beyond the limits of their capabilities, pushed beyond their physical strength, so that all they can do is weep bitter tears of frustration. Even Jesus wept over Jerusalem, knowing that His tender care for it would be rejected.

At times, each one of us will cry as the psalmist did: "Out of the depths I cry to you, O Lord!" (Ps 130:1, NRSVCE). Yet, even our tears can be redemptive.

October 28

Feast of Saints Simon and Jude

Why Did You Reveal Yourself to Us?

"The one thing that she [Our Lady] did and does is the one thing that we all have to do, namely, to bear Christ into the world."

— Caryll Houselander, *The Reed of God*

Saint Simon is known as "the zealot," and Saint Jude Thaddeus is the one who asked Jesus at the Last Supper, "Why did you reveal yourself to us and not to the whole world?" Because, of course, we know that if He wanted to do so, He could have. He might have revealed himself in a blinding flash of unmistakable power and glory, from one end of the heavens to the other. So Jesus answered him, "Whoever loves me will keep my word, and my Father will love him, and we will come to him and make our dwelling with him" (Jn 14:23).

When God dwells within us — when He lives in our hearts — then we will be able to take Him to everyone we meet. Then He will be revealed to the rest of the world.

October 29

Heavy Doors

"After this I had a vision of an open door to heaven."

— Revelation 4:1

It takes a lot of maneuvering to get through the steel doors. First, you enter the code, wait for the green light, push open the heavy door with your backside, then back the wheelchair out . . . all this before the alarm goes off. At last, we breathe in the scent of honeysuckle and sunshine.

Like these heavy doors, the gate to eternal life is not easy to get through. Jesus describes it as "narrow" (Mt 7:14). The door of heaven beckons us into a garden where the breeze blows cool in the afternoon. It is delicately scented with the incense of heavenly hosannas, offering true joy in the light of the Lamb. Jesus himself opens this door.

OCTOBER 30

Worth Remembering

"'Dr. Snowdon, do you know what my worst fear was?' Now her eyes started to well up with tears. 'That I was going to forget Jesus,' she said. 'I finally realized that I may not remember Him, but He will remember me.'"

— David Snowdon, *Aging With Grace*

By the year 2025, it is estimated that there will be 7 million people suffering from Alzheimer's. A sixty-eight-year-old retired physician recently began blogging about his own diagnosis. He hopes to counter the fear and embarrassment surrounding the disease by openly discussing his symptoms and his life journey. He writes that, so far, he is happier than he used to be. He is more vulnerable and open to others. Yet, he fears the loneliness and isolation that the advanced stages of the disease may bring. He hopes to prevent that by sharing what it's like, from the inside.

October 31

Dry Bones

"Faith is linked to hope, for even if our dwelling place here below is wasting away, we have an eternal dwelling place which God has already prepared in Christ, in his body."

— Pope Francis, *Lumen Fidei*

The prophet Ezekiel had a vision of a vast plain filled with dry bones. God told him to prophesy over the bones: "Dry bones, hear the word of the Lord!" (Ez 37:4). You can picture the scene: storm clouds roiling above a gray wasteland of rattling bones coming to life, like a zombie apocalypse.

How often do the elderly feel like Ezekiel's dry bones? They groan, "Our bones are dried up, our hope is lost." But just as in the Old Testament vision, God will breathe His spirit into them. He will raise them up and bring them to everlasting life. Hope is not lost!

November 1

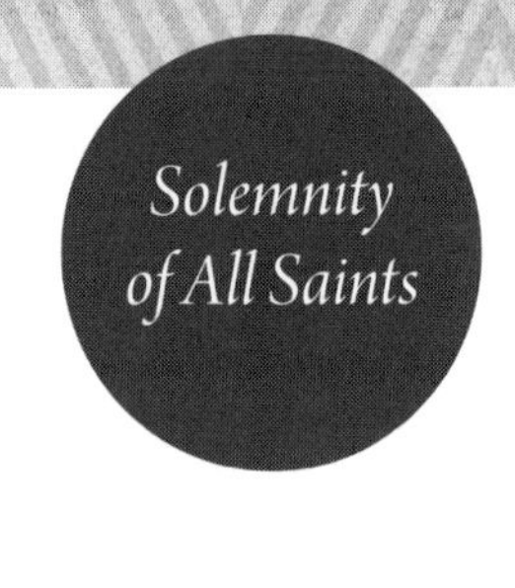

Dancing with the (Real) Stars

"Oh Lord, I want to be in that number when the saints go marching in."

— Traditional Spiritual

"In the saints we see the victory of love over selfishness and death: we see that following Christ leads to life, eternal life, and gives meaning to the present, every moment that passes, because it is filled with love and hope."

— Pope Benedict XVI, *Angelus,* November 1, 2012

I push my mom in her wheelchair into the front lobby. We are surprised by live music, balloons, and tables of happy residents. It's one gentleman's ninety-and-a-half birthday and he's got a conga line going as the band plays *When the Saints Go Marching In*. Everyone — in their wheelchairs, with their walkers, or carrying a cane — is dancing. My mom laughs, a blessed sound. God surprises us with His grace. Saints in the making!

NOVEMBER 2

Never Too Late

"In the interconnectedness of Being, my gratitude to the other — my prayer for him — can play a small part in his purification. And for that there is no need to convert earthly time into God's time: in the communion of souls simple terrestrial time is superseded. It is never too late to touch the heart of another, nor is it ever in vain."

— Pope Benedict XVI, *Spe Salvi*

A woman in our parish committed suicide. Nobody had an inkling that her emotional state was so desperate and that she would take her own life. Many prayers and Masses were offered. There were prayers from hundreds of people who wished, for example, that they had said something uplifting that day they ran into her at Starbucks. Others wished they had stopped to talk to her after morning Mass that day she seemed a bit upset. Can we apologize now for our insensitivity, for those times we ignored her, assuming she had it all together? Will our prayers help? In God's time, yes. God's time is *kairos*, the eternal present. It encompasses all time, but is not constricted by it. It's never too late to reach out.

NOVEMBER 3

Be Not Crushed

"Be not crushed on their account, as though I would leave you crushed before them; For it is I this day who have made you a fortified city, A pillar of iron, a wall of brass, against the whole land: Against Judah's kings and princes, against its priests and people. They will fight against you, but not prevail over you, for I am with you to deliver you, says the LORD."

— Jeremiah 1:17-19, NAB

We often hear the advice "Be not afraid." But, when we are dealing every day with the physical frailties of our loved ones and our own physical weakness and ever-growing weariness, we need to hear "Be not *crushed!*" You are a fortified city, a pillar of iron, a wall of brass. Oh, you may not feel like it, not today, when your back is aching and you've got the mother-of-all-headaches. But let's remember that God tells us He has done everything for us. And then we can stand strong.

November 4

The Lord Looks into the Heart

"God does not see as a mortal, who sees the appearance. The Lord looks into the heart."

— 1 Samuel 16:7

My friend's daughter, Janie, is slightly learning disabled. Nonetheless, she has a clear vision of what she wants to do in life. She loves to serve the elderly. So many of us today turn our faces away from the suffering, the poor, the handicapped, and the otherwise unattractive. We look to magazines, fashion models, and TV instead. But, the pure of heart will see God. Janie sees God in every elderly person she serves, and her face is alight with joy.

NOVEMBER 5

Reverse Mission

"Jesus did not say: 'Blessed are those who care for the poor,' but 'Blessed are the poor.' Simple as this remark may seem, it offers the key to the kingdom."

— Henri Nouwen, *Here and Now*

When Henri Nouwen first began working with the residents at L'Arche, a faith-based community of friendship and support for the intellectually disabled, he thought he was going there to help them. He quickly discovered God's "reverse mission": "I soon learned that my real task would be to let those whom I wanted to help offer me — and through me many others — their unique spiritual gifts."

The sick help us heal, and the dying help us live.

November 6

Carrying Your Father

"Christian patience . . . is the patience of Saint Paul, which means enduring, bearing history on one's shoulders. It's the archetypal image of Aeneas, who, as Troy burned, took his father on his shoulders . . . took his history on his shoulders and walked toward the mountain in search of the future."

— Pope Francis, *Conversations with Jorge Bergoglio: His Life in His Own Words*

As Troy burns, Aeneas escapes with his young son, carrying his elderly father on his shoulders. The image strikes a chord with me, reminding me that we baby boomers, like Aeneas, are responsible for both young and old. We are the "sandwich" generation. While attending to our immediate family (spouse and children), we are also caring for our aging parents. Rather than thinking of this as a burden, isn't it far more beautiful to think of it in terms of Christian patience?

November 7

Transforming Hearts

"There are few things that bring greater balm and peace to the soul than to bring them to the soul of another."

— Gerald Vann, O.P., *The Seven Sweet Blessings of Christ*

Fifty-two million Americans care for a loved one with a disability or serious medical condition. One of these is Becky, who cares for her husband who suffers from MS. He's in a wheelchair, and can do nothing for himself. Becky rises at five in the morning to get him ready for the day before she goes to work.

Another is the father of Dominic, the young boy with cerebral palsy whom Pope Francis famously embraced on Easter Sunday 2013. Dominic's father writes about Dominic's suffering and about his own, as a caregiver who must help him every moment of every day. Why does God allow such suffering, especially of the innocent? The answer, says Dominic's dad, is so we can learn to love. So our stony hearts will turn into hearts of compassion, like the heart of Jesus.

November 8

Divine Mystery in Things

"Love a man even in his sin, for that is the semblance of Divine Love and is the highest love on earth. Love all God's creation, the whole and every grain of sand in it. Love every leaf, every ray of God's light. Love the animals, love the plants, love everything. If you love everything, you will perceive the divine mystery in things."

— Fyodor Dostoyevsky, *The Brothers Karamazov*

Abraham was sitting under the terebinth of Mamre, at the entrance of his tent, as the day was growing hot. He saw three men and immediately he invited them in for a special meal. If Abraham had not glimpsed something important — if he had not seen the supernatural possibility in his ordinary life on that hot afternoon, if he had not invited the men to stay for a meal — Sarah might not have conceived and Abraham might not be our father in faith. He would not have discovered hope (see Gn 18).

Tiny Nellie sits every morning, before the day grows hot, under the great oak branches on "her" little bench. She sits serenely looking out over the meadow. Her daily meditation under the spreading branches keeps her in touch with the divine mystery in things.

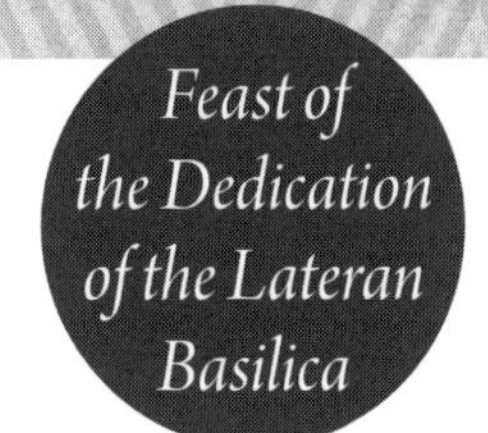

November 9

Living Stones

"Come to him, a living stone, rejected by human beings but chosen and precious in the eyes of God, and, like living stones, let yourselves be built into a spiritual house."

— 1 Peter 2:4-5

Some theologians say that sacred space (like a church or a tabernacle or a mosque) is a physical space that mediates between appearance and reality. The truly real is unseen, like the interior of the holy of holies, or God in the burning bush, or Jesus at the moment of transubstantiation. The nursing home is sacred space, too. Within its walls are suffering holy ones, men and women whose appearance belies their sacred worth. They are themselves tabernacles of Jesus.

NOVEMBER 10

Sharing

"The community of believers was of one heart and mind, and no one claimed that any of his possessions was his own, but they had everything in common."

— Acts 4:32

The early Christians didn't need to possess many things. They had the joy of the risen Lord in their hearts. I reluctantly gave someone the wind chime that I had previously given my parents for their deck. She promised to take good care of it and told me that it's going to a home where it will be cherished. I want all of these things for myself, but it's better to share them.

November 11

Feast of Saint Martin of Tours, Veterans Day

Strength for the Daily Battle

"I was . . . naked and you clothed me."

— Matthew 25:35-36

Saint Martin of Tours, born in the early fourth century, is an icon of Christian charity. He was a soldier and a catechumen — he had become a catechumen at the age of ten, against his pagan parent's wishes. He was still unbaptized when he had a mysterious encounter with a poor man. One night, while coming through the city gates, he met a man dressed in rags, freezing in the crisp air. Martin stopped, cut his cloak in two with his sword, and gave half to the stranger. Later that night, Jesus appeared to him in a dream, wearing the cloak. Deeply moved, Martin immediately went off to be baptized. He spent the rest of his life in service to the Lord.

Saint Martin is the patron saint of soldiers, and today we honor him along with the veterans who sacrificially and heroically fought for the sake of freedom. Let us pray that God does not hide His face, but gives them, as well as the elderly and infirm, strength to see Him in the midst of suffering.

November 12

Sacred Time

"On the watchtower, my Lord,

I stand constantly by day;

And I stay at my post

through all the watches of the night."

— Isaiah 21:8

It's three in the morning in the darkened abbey, and the hooded monks intone slowly, gravely: "For my days vanish like smoke; my bones burn away as in a furnace" (Ps 102:4)

They are few, these holy men, these night watchmen for Christ and His coming. Five of them are able-bodied, two with walkers, several stooped with age. The youngest is in his fifties. They file slowly, silently, out of the chapel. Every hour, every moment of every day is consecrated to God. The psalm prayers waft heavenward like incense. This must be what it means to *pray without ceasing.*

November 13

One Last Time

"The belief that love can reach into the afterlife, that reciprocal giving and receiving is possible. . . . Who would not feel the need to convey to their departed loved ones a sign of kindness, a gesture of gratitude or even a request for pardon?"

— Pope Benedict XVI, *Spe Salvi*

My dad died before I was ready. Perhaps everyone feels this way about a loved one's passing. I didn't get a chance to ask him to play his harmonica one last time. I didn't ask him to tell me about the Chosin Reservoir, one of the deadliest battles of the Korean War, one last time. I didn't tell him I loved him one last time. The words unsaid, the time not spent. Today, at the nursing home, we are serenaded by a man with a hammered dulcimer singing *Down in the Valley.* It was one of my dad's favorite harmonica tunes. My mom's eyes light up. "Angels in Heaven know I love you; know I love you, dear, know I love you." Love reaches into the afterlife.

November 14

Hiddenness

"A waiting person is a patient person. The word 'patience' means the willingness to stay where we are and live the situation out to the full in the belief that something hidden there will manifest itself to us."

— *Mornings with Henri Nouwen*

When the seed goes into the dark, deep earth, it lays there, hidden, for a time. It seems as though nothing is happening, but that is only from the perspective of the surface. Unseen roots are generating, hidden miracles are at work. It's the same with those suffering in silence. They are waiting while the invisible is at work, generating their new life. There is nothing hidden that will not be revealed.

NOVEMBER 15

The Dwelling

"The one who stayed with us in the past and will return to us in the future becomes present to us in that precious moment in which memory and hope touch each other."

— *Mornings with Henri Nouwen*

There's a mysterious thing that happens when you love someone. When you love someone, and he is in the house, you feel his presence. When he is gone, you feel his presence — as absence — even more. You long for him, you wait up for him, you feel more alone without him. When I went home after my dad died, I thought I heard his voice. "Hi, hi!" he would say as soon as I walked in the door. Now the house is empty, so empty. Yet I believe, because Jesus tells me, that my dad still lives.

November 16

The Offering of Ourselves

"We are often surprised when, after we have offered God several litanies a day, and a pest of little mortifications, He chooses instead something that is really ourselves; our solitude for example, or the sweetness of the feeling of love; or, as is very frequent now, our home. It is what God chooses that kindles in the crucible and burns the flame of love."

— Caryll Houselander, *The Passion of the Infant Christ*

What pleases God? It can be a daily commute to work, a gentle touch, a kind word, the time you didn't snap at your kids, silence when you'd rather argue, your caregiving. All of these, and so many more simple things, done out of love.

November 17

Empty-handed

"For we brought nothing into the world, just as we shall not be able to take anything out of it."

— 1 Timothy 6:7, NAB

Our very elderly priest shuffles slowly to the altar, wheezing. Nonetheless, his voice is strong. He says we can't bring anything with us when we die. We depart as we come into this world. Taking care of elderly loved ones is a poignant reminder of this. Then, why does Ben Sira (the Book of Sirach) tell us, "Do not appear before the Lord empty-handed" (35:6)?

What can we carry past the dark night of the final loneliness, past the grave so we are not empty-handed? Perhaps only a heart filled with love for our friends and family, our hands open, not grasping, with our love freely given?

November 18

Power of Love

"In this way the love of God was revealed to us: God sent his only Son into the world so that we might have life through him. In this is love: not that we have loved God, but that he loved us."

— 1 John 4:9-10

Today Mrs. X. is a new woman. Beaming, eyes sparkling, she introduces me to her daughter, who flew across the country for a surprise visit! This is the good news of salvation. He has come to heal the brokenhearted! Today, everyone is given a reprieve. There is no berating or chastising of nurses, residents, and visitors. Today, there are no sullen looks or impossible demands. Here is proof of the transformational power of love. In being loved, she can love. Is it any wonder that God is love?

November 19

God's Grip

"Hold fast to Christ; he carries you through the night of death that he himself has overcome."

— Cardinal Joseph Ratzinger, *Images of Hope*

Jacob stayed up all night, wrestling with a mysterious stranger. At dawn, the stranger told him to let him go, but Jacob refused to let him go and demanded a blessing (see Gn 32:25-30). Sometimes, we have to wrestle with God, with His mysterious ways. We can bring our struggles, our frustrations, and our complaints to prayer, and insist on God's blessing.

Sometimes, my mom refuses to let us take her out of bed, but we know it is better for her. And in the end, when she is able to go outside and enjoy the flower gardens, she appreciates the effort. Don't let grace slip away without a struggle.

November 20

He Is Deeper Still

"'We must tell them that there is no pit so deep that He is not deeper still. They will listen to us, Corrie, because we have been here.'"

— Corrie Ten Boom, *The Hiding Place*

Corrie and her sister Betsie were imprisoned at Ravensbruck concentration camp for helping Jews escape the Nazis in Holland. They were brutally handled at the camp, packed into squalid rooms, mocked and beaten by Nazi guards. Through it all, Betsie prayed for her persecutors. She thanked God for everything — even the fleas. Corrie (who thought Betsie was over the top) later discovered that because of their flea-infested prison room, their group had remained unguarded. They had the freedom to read the Bible, pray, and sing hymns every day. Though Betsie died in the concentration camp, Corrie survived. She was able to bring the message of God's hope and mercy to generations worldwide. At Ravensbruck, they had learned that Christ's love can transform even the darkest pit of human despair.

NOVEMBER 21

Transforming Suffering

"It is not by sidestepping or fleeing from suffering that we are healed, but rather by our capacity for accepting it, maturing through it and finding meaning through union with Christ, who suffered with infinite love."

— Pope Benedict XVI, *Spe Salvi*

Though Jesus healed the sick, He didn't heal everyone who was sick. Similarly, the *Catechism of the Catholic Church* reminds us that "even the most intense prayers" (1508) do not always result in healing. Christ entered this world, taking on our own afflictions, experiencing pain and suffering himself. He came not to eradicate every suffering, but to transform it.

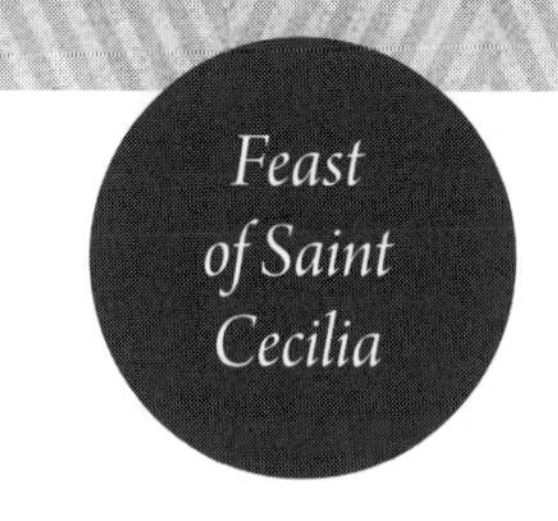

NOVEMBER 22

Singing to God in Your Heart

"While the instruments were playing, she sang to God in her heart."

— Cardinal Joseph Ratzinger, *Co-Workers of the Truth*

The patron saint of music, Saint Cecilia chose the eternal music of the heavenly hosts, rather than the instruments of the world. She and all the saints continue to sing eternally before the glory of God in heaven. We, too, hope to be, in some way, God's instruments in this world. We hope to do His will and proclaim His saving power.

Legend has it that Cecilia, though she had taken a vow of virginity, was forced to marry a young Roman. She converted him to Christianity and he was subsequently martyred. She herself was condemned to suffocation (which failed). Later, an executioner attempted unsuccessfully to decapitate the saint, three times. Though the stories of the numerous attempts on her life are considered to be pious legend, the fact that she sang to God in her heart rings true.

November 23

The Cloud of Unknowing

"Having a cloud in the brain that throbs with 'It's bad to be me' is not a sin. The cloud is a distortion in self-consciousness based in a physical disorder and aggravated by external circumstances. The central temptation of the devil is his attempt to convince us, 'It is bad to be you! And it's your fault!' This is a big lie."

— John Janaro, *Never Give Up*

God spoke to Moses from within a burning bush, but also from a heavy cloud over Mount Sinai (see Ex 19:9). The cloud is the sacred sign of God's hidden presence. An anonymous mystic wrote a book on contemplative prayer called *The Cloud of Unknowing.* When we are striving to hear God's voice or to discern His will, it often seems that He is wrapped in a dense cloud. And, sometimes, we cannot hear Him at all. This is the time of dark faith, when we are in the midst of the cloud of unknowing. We have nothing to go on, neither reason nor feeling, but simply trust.

November 24

The Wisdom of Age

"Two weeks before her ninetieth birthday, Sister Genevieve Kunkel marveled at her well-being. 'I have two good traits,' she told me. 'I am alert and I am vertical.'"

— David Snowdon, *Aging with Grace*

When Joshua was "old and advanced in years," he called all the people of Israel together and recounted the marvelous things God had done for them. He began with Abraham and Moses in the desert, sharing how God brought them out of slavery and protected them on their journey. Then, Joshua died at the age of one hundred ten (see Jos 24:1-30).

We, too, as we grow older, should recount God's blessings for our families and those we care for. Sometimes, it can be difficult to find the blessings in the day to day. But, even our life itself is a gift! Joshua reminds us to be continually thankful for God's many blessings — even up to the end of our lives.

November 25

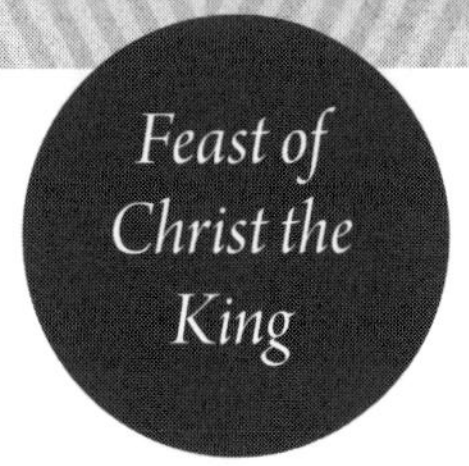

God's Kingship

"This, then, is God's kingship — a rule of love that seeks and finds man in ways that are always new. . . . God can always be found. The pattern of our own lives should also be like this — we should always be available, never write anyone off, and try again and again to find others in the openness of our hearts . . . always to be ready to set off on the way to God and to each other."

— Pope Benedict XVI, *Seeking God's Face*

The tiny human being at conception, with all his genetic code in place; the silent suffering of the abandoned elderly; the older child, no longer a sweet baby, passed over again for adoption; the dark-skinned men who wait, huddled together outside 7-Eleven, hoping someone will choose them to work today. God waits, silent, for us to find Him.

November 26

Human Beings, Not Doings

"Before all else, we need to keep alive in our world the thirst for the absolute, and to counter the dominance of a one-dimensional vision of the human person, a vision that reduces human beings to what they produce and to what they consume."

— Pope Francis, *Address,* March 20, 2013

Why do we always feel that we must be *doing* something, being productive, moving forward? The world values us for what we do, for what we accomplish. But this doesn't count as much in the eyes of God. From the smallest babe to the octogenarian, we are precious to Him. We need to learn to be still. "Be still and know that I am God!" says the Lord. He can only be heard when we are still, when we are not busy *doing*, but simply *being* (see Ps 46:11).

NOVEMBER 27

Healing Icon

"You answer every petition, alleviate sorrows, grant health to the ailing, heal the weak and ill, drive away the demons from the possessed, deliver the offended from misfortune, cleanse the impure and have mercy upon little children: moreover, O Mistress Lady Theotokos, you free from chains the imprisoned and heal all manner of passions. For everything is possible by your intercession before your Son, Christ our God."

— Prayer to the Most Holy Theotokos, Healer

After my mom's stroke, I picked up a beautiful Russian icon at the Shrine of the Immaculate Conception for my mom's hospital room. The Blessed Mother, wearing a crown, stands by the bedside of a sick man, a scepter poised in her left hand. I asked a friend who lives in Moscow to translate the words on the back. She told me that the icon is of a miraculous image of the Theotokos (meaning Mother of God), Healer. The image relates the story of a miraculous healing of a Russian priest who had prayed daily to the Theotokos. In turn, many who prayed in front of the icon were healed. Who has more compassion for a sick child than a mother?

NOVEMBER 28

Seeing with the Eyes of Your Heart

"I love what Job says after his difficult experience and the dialogues that did not help him in any way: 'By hearsay I had heard of you, but now my eye has seen you.' What I tell people is not to know God only by hearing. The Living God is He that you may see with your eyes within your heart."

— Cardinal Jorge Mario Bergoglio, *On Heaven and Earth*

Do you see the face of God in your heart? The great mystic Saint Teresa of Avila tells us that our soul is the interior castle in which God dwells, and prayer is the door. Yet, how often we spend our days distractedly roaming around outside the castle walls. In fact, we spend so much time outside the castle that we forget it's even there. The entryway becomes overgrown with ivy and thorn bushes. We no longer remember how to enter our own heart. Let's put aside the many distractions, the to-do list that insistently calls us. Leave behind the thorns of worldly anxiety, and instead enter the castle in our hearts.

November 29

Stay Awake

"The Bridegroom is the Lord, and the time of waiting for his arrival is the time he gives to us, to all of us, before his Final Coming with mercy and patience; it is a time of watchfulness; a time in which we must keep alight the lamps of faith, hope and charity. . . . What he asks of us is to be ready for the encounter — ready for an encounter, for a beautiful encounter, the encounter with Jesus."

— Pope Francis, *General Audience*, April 24, 2013

The long-delayed bridegroom comes while all the virgins in the wedding party have become drowsy. When the cry is sounded at midnight, the five foolish ones must leave to purchase more oil (see Mt 25:1-13). Some Scripture scholars say that this oil is the oil of the sacraments, especially the sacrament of forgiveness and mercy, which prepares us to meet Jesus without stain of sin. Others say that the oil is that of good works and charity. In any case, at that hour, there is no more time to do good works or to seek forgiveness.

Father anoints my mom with sacred chrism oil on her forehead and her hands. I hold her hand gently, as she waits in silence for the herald angel, for the sound of the distant trumpet to call her home.

NOVEMBER 30

Feast of Saint Andrew

At Once They Followed Him

"As [Jesus] was walking by the Sea of Galilee, he saw two brothers, Simon who is called Peter, and his brother Andrew, casting a net into the sea; they were fishermen. He said to them, 'Come after me, and I will make you fishers of men.' At once they left their nets and followed him."

— Matthew 4:18-20

These two fishermen probably had no clue what Jesus meant when He said He would make them fishers of men. They probably thought it sounded strange and mysterious, certainly not the plain speech they were used to as fishermen. They dropped what they were doing and immediately followed Him, because they had been watching and waiting for the coming of the Messiah. They knew there was something more to life than the workday — heading out on water, lowering nets, waiting for a catch and hauling it in, heading back to shore, repairing nets. They had been waiting, longing for the one who would give meaning to their lives, give them hope for the future, assure them that they had a mission to accomplish.

DECEMBER 1

Waiting

"And God himself will be with them; he will wipe every tear from their eyes."

— Revelation 21:3-4, NRSVCE

Small children wait in eager anticipation for Christmas. For them, waiting is almost the best part. But we adults are always in a hurry to move to the next level, to finish a project, get a degree, get married, be successful. We don't always see the beauty of the waiting, especially if it is accompanied by illness. And for those in the nursing home, there is nothing *but* the waiting. Yet, for the one who believes, waiting is neither meaningless nor tiresome. Every moment holds meaning, pregnant with hope. Donna is holding hands with an elderly gentleman, also from the Alzheimer's unit. "Are you two going out?" I tease. She laughs delightedly, like a young girl.

December 2

A Word in Waiting

"I believe that in our own day . . . we can share anew this sense of astonishment at the fact that a saying from the year 733 B.C., incomprehensible for so long, came true at the moment of the conception of Jesus Christ — that God did indeed give us a great sign intended for the whole world."

— Pope Benedict XVI, *Jesus of Nazareth*

When Isaiah spoke about the coming of Immanuel, God-with-us, there was no precedent for this word and no historical basis. "The Lord himself will give you a sign. Behold, a virgin shall conceive and bear a son, and shall call his name Immanuel" (Is 7:14, RSVCE). He was not prophesying about Hezekiah, the son of King Ahaz, or about one of his own sons. He wasn't even talking about Israel itself. It was, as Pope Benedict says, a "word in waiting." It was a mystery at the time and to the prophet himself.

We each have a word in waiting, spoken to us by God in the depths of our hearts.

December 3

Signs of Love

"The tree at Christkindl . . . is at the same time a monstrance, the appearance of the One who is the bread of life, the appearance of salvation. And this tree is a cross — and thus has become an altar. The child bears the cross and the crown of thorns in his hands. These are the signs of the love that transforms the tree into a cross and the cross into the table of life."

— Cardinal Joseph Ratzinger, *The Blessing of Christmas*

The oldest surviving Christmas tree is enshrined in a church in Germany. In fact, the church was built around the tree! In a hollow of this tree is a miraculous image of the Christ Child, placed there by a pious choirmaster back in the 1600s. The man had a "falling down" illness, perhaps epilepsy, and used to pray before this tree.

Cardinal Joseph Ratzinger visited the Christkindl church and wrote about his experience there. As he said, we all suffer from a falling-down sickness. We need Christ's help to get through life. The tree with its twinkling fairy lights that I place in my mom's room might not be miraculous, but I know it offers a ray of hope.

December 4

A Visit from the Lord

"Just like a great joy, so too illness and suffering can be a very personal Advent of one's own — a visit by the God who enters my life and wants to encounter me personally."

— Cardinal Joseph Ratzinger, *The Blessing of Christmas*

During the month of December, we are often so busy preparing for guests, buying Christmas presents, cooking and cleaning, that we forget to prepare for Christ's birth. Sometimes, we have so many pressing things to deal with that we can't even take a moment to reflect on God's word spoken in the silence of our hearts.

But the one who is ill, confined to bed, sometimes alone and in pain, is visited by God in a different way. God speaks to the person in the waiting, through the pain, in the forced confinement of the sickbed. God speaks a word of hope. He is coming as the infant Jesus.

DECEMBER 5

A Journeying Faith

"The darkness of faith is just as pleasing to God as the consolations of faith. In fact, the darkness of faith is what prunes you, detaches you, and makes you love God with a pure love."

— *Mother Angelica's Private and Pithy Lessons from Scripture*

There are days when we don't see God's purpose in our lives, and everything seems dark. We don't have a clue about where we are going or what the next step is supposed to be. Pope Benedict XVI wrote that even Mary did not always understand the purpose of certain events, or what Jesus was telling her. Her faith was a "journeying" faith, sometimes "shrouded in darkness." On those days when you simply can't see what the next step should be, ask the Blessed Mother to hold your hand. Ask her to lead you through the darkness. Become like a trusting child.

DECEMBER 6

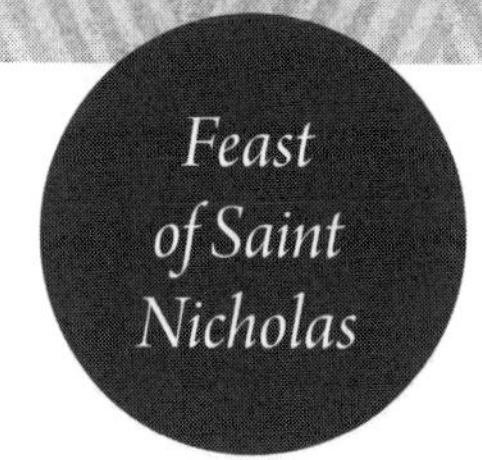

Gift

"Once I only thanked Santa Claus for a few dolls and crackers, now, I thank him for stars and street faces, and wine and the great sea."

— G.K. Chesterton

I used to put chocolate candy in my kids' shoes to celebrate this feast day. Now my kids are grown, but I do have my mom. I wonder whether I might sneak some chocolate to my mom today. Perhaps something especially soft and melty, like a creamy truffle. She's not allowed to eat because of swallowing difficulties. We insist on Holy Communion, however. And I'm thinking: why not chocolate, too?

Caring for the elderly or sick helps us appreciate the small and simple things of life that, when we are busy and active, are often overlooked. We can thank Him for the stars overhead, the fact that we can see the stars, that first bite of chocolate, the Lord on our tongue. All are gifts from God.

December 7

Dreaming the Future

"Such was his intention when, behold, the angel of the Lord appeared to him in a dream and said, 'Joseph, son of David, do not be afraid.'"

— Matthew 1:20

I dreamed last night about my dad. He was young, about thirty, and so handsome. He and my mom, also young, jumped in their old Chevy. Mom was wearing a shirtwaist dress that gaily billowed out. Perhaps, through my dream, my dad is consoling me from heaven. One day he and my mom will be alive together, young again. Eternally happy.

December 8

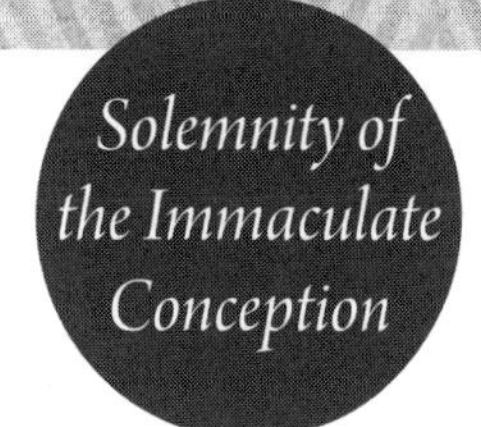

Perfectly Centered in God

"This is the result of [Mary] being without original sin: her relationship with God is free of even [the] smallest cracks; there is no separation, there is no shadow of egoism, only perfect harmony: her little human heart is perfectly "centered" in the great heart of God."

— Pope Benedict XVI, *Address on the Feast of the Immaculate Conception*, 2012

From the moment of conception in her mother's womb, Mary is filled with the grace of God. Throughout her life, nothing separates her from God the Father — no selfish desire, no self-centered thought. She is always quick to respond to the needs of her family and friends, her neighbors. She travels in haste to visit Elizabeth as soon as she hears the news of her elderly cousin's pregnancy. We can imagine her bringing meals to neighbors, helping with chores, listening to the Word of God at the synagogue. She is gentle and kind, filled with joy and laughter, open to love. Yet, she is not a statue. She is a real human being with free will. Her little human heart beats to the rhythm of God's great heart.

DECEMBER 9

God's Warmth

"Warmed by the signs, we can then receive in full confidence the immeasurable kindness of this child who alone had the power to make the mountains sing and to transform the trees of the wood into a praise of God."

— Cardinal Joseph Ratzinger, *The Blessing of Christmas*

I take my mom upstairs to the lobby to view the huge Christmas tree that dominates the entrance. It has giant balls that even the nearly blind can spot from a distance. The residents who are able help decorate. The tree's bottom branches are at the perfect height for someone in a wheelchair. Then, back in her room, I decorate a small tree with glistening lights, reminding us of Christ's love that dispels even the darkest night.

DECEMBER 10

God Is Close

"God is not some remote highest being, forever inaccessible. He is very close to us; we can call to him; we can always reach him. He has time for me."

— Cardinal Joseph Ratzinger, *The Blessing of Christmas*

The coming of Jesus into the world overturns all previous ideas about God. No longer is salvation only for the wealthy, the smart, and the powerful. God comes *first* to the shepherds, the animals in the stable, the poor and the ignorant. He comes as a tiny babe. Even the youngest child can hold an infant in his arms.

December 11

Patient Servant

"Be patient and show in every way that you are servants of God. Say: And now, what do I wait for? Is it not the Lord?"

— Origen, *Exhortation to Martyrdom*

It's a snowy day in Washington, D.C., when Mary's daughter Courtney has a doctor's appointment downtown. As Mary hunts for a parking place for the giant handicapped-equipped van on the busy downtown street, Courtney has a major seizure. Yet, Mary maintains her positive attitude and goes with the flow.

How do I react when things don't go my way? I pout and complain! Yet, isn't it in moments like these when I might work on holiness? I don't have to get my eyes gouged out like Saint Lucy, or be shot full of arrows like Saint Sebastian, or pressed to death like Saint Margaret Clitherow. I might, instead, accept setbacks and frustrations with humility.

December 12

Feast of Our Lady of Guadalupe

Secret Garden

"In [Our Lady] the Word of God chose to be silent for the season measured by God. She, too, was silent; in her the light of the world shone in darkness. Today, in many souls, Christ asks that He may grow secretly, that He may be the light shining in the darkness."

— Caryll Houselander, *The Reed of God*

How much of God's life in the world is hidden, secret?

December 13

Immovable Faith

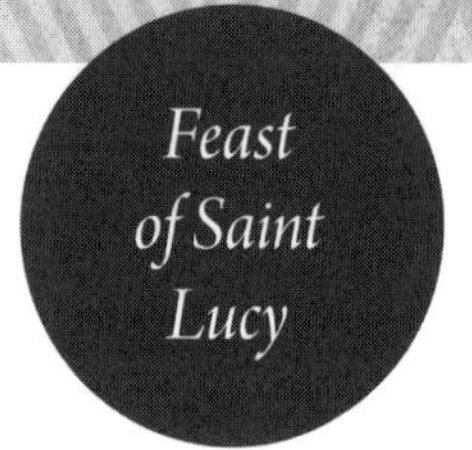

"Be firm, steadfast, always fully devoted to the work of the Lord, knowing that in the Lord your labor is not in vain."

— 1 Corinthians 15: 58

The Italian painter Lorenzo Lotto created an altarpiece that depicts Saint Lucy, a beautiful young girl with pink cheeks, standing fearlessly before the Roman consul. She is dressed in a bright yellow gown, defiantly pointing to heaven. She faces the incredulous Paschasius who sentences her to a brothel because she refuses to marry. She has promised her life to Christ. The people around her are trying to drag her away, but they can't. She does not budge; she's immovable.

Let's pray that we, too, can hold fast to our faith, fearless in the face of evil.

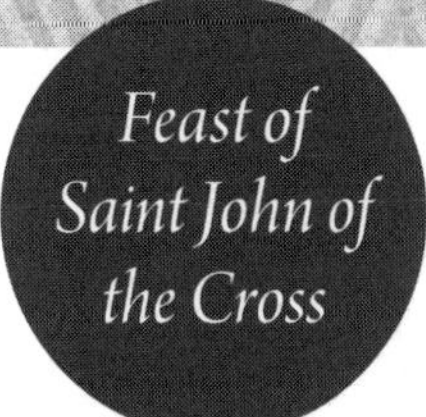

DECEMBER 14

Where There Is No Love, Put Love

"At the evening of life, we shall be judged on our love."

— Saint John of the Cross, *Prologue to the Ascent of Mount Carmel*

Saint John of the Cross was a Carmelite mystic and poet who, together with Saint Teresa of Avila, led a reform movement of the order. He was imprisoned by his own monks in a nine-by-five-foot hole in the wall with no window He was beaten three times a day so severely that he bore scars. After nine months of this torture and imprisonment, he finally managed a dramatic escape. Yet he never became embittered or discouraged. Instead, he wrote: "Think nothing else but that God ordains all, and where there is no love, put love, and you will draw out love."

Caregivers often suffer a dark night, as do our loved ones who are imprisoned by sickbeds or the four walls of their sickrooms. Let our prayer, like Saint John's, be our light in the darkness. And may we put love wherever there is none.

DECEMBER 15

Incarnation

"On that Holy Night, in taking flesh God wanted to make a gift of himself to men and women, he gave himself for us; God made his Only Son a gift for us, he took on our humanity to give his divinity to us. This is the great gift."

— Pope Benedict XVI, *General Audience*, January 9, 2013

What does the Incarnation mean for us, really? Say, on an average Wednesday afternoon? What does it mean that God — creator and upholder of all things, the infinite and eternal Being himself — became a particular human person, born at a particular time in history? Does it mean, perhaps, that God wanted to be part of our lives in a much more radically intimate way? Does it mean, perhaps, that there is something about God incarnated into every aspect of human existence? Does it mean that He knows us from the inside, and wishes to meet us there?

DECEMBER 16

You Are a Star!

"To look at the star means receiving light and giving light, radiating in the world around us the light that we have received, so that it can provide orientation to others, too. . . . Once our heart has awakened, we see around us so many others who are waiting for a light. Let them not call out to us in vain."

— Cardinal Joseph Ratzinger, *The Blessing of Christmas*

The star that guided the Magi to adore the Christ Child is today the star of our faith, and the star of our friends in Christ. Our faith and our friends keep us traveling east, toward the true light. When our kids were very small, we carried candles and sang Christmas carols as we strolled through the neighborhood. We were lights for each other and for the world, for the ones who don't know Him yet. Each day, you bring your light to the one for whom you care. You are the light that lights up the darkness of loneliness and illness.

DECEMBER 17

O Wisdom

"O Wisdom, O holy Word of God, you govern all creation with your strong yet tender care. Come and show your people the way to salvation."

— *O Antiphon for Advent Vespers*

Beginning on December 17, during the Octave before Christmas, we recite the "O antiphons" during the evening prayers of the Church. Each of the antiphons contains a title of the Messiah and refers us to Isaiah's prophesy about the coming of the Messiah (see Is 11:2-3; 28:29). Today, it is "O Sapientia," "O Wisdom," for Isaiah said that the spirit of wisdom would rest on the Messiah.

Let us pray today for wisdom in caring for our loved ones and for ourselves. Pray that we will know and be able to provide what we all need, physically and spiritually.

DECEMBER 18

O Adonai

"O sacred Lord of ancient Israel, who showed yourself to Moses in the burning bush, who gave him the holy law on Sinai mountain: come, stretch out your mighty hand to set us free."

— *O Antiphon for Advent Vespers*

This sacred Lord, the Lord of the burning bush, the very same creator of the universe, humbles himself to be planted as though He were a tiny seedling, in His mother's womb. He grew, silently, slowly, hidden, the way of all babies. The message for us today is that this time and this space is sacred. The way of joy must come through the way of waiting, of darkness, of smallness. A caregiver's life is often just this way, too. But the smallness, the humility of the work, the silence of the waiting . . . will end in joy.

December 19

O Radix Jesse

"O Flower of Jesse's stem, you have been raised up as a sign for all peoples; kings stand silent in your presence; the nations bow down in worship before you. Come, let nothing keep you from coming to our aid."

— *O Antiphon for Advent Vespers*

Unable to walk, Irene was in bed, waiting for news of the seedlings her son had planted for her. "Do you have any good news?" she asked, after I returned from my check on the flower boxes. We are surprised and thrilled when the flowers burst forth.

The prophet Isaiah foretold that "a shoot shall sprout from the stump of Jesse, and from his roots a bud shall blossom" (Is 11:1). The bud is Our Lord, who was born into the family of King David, the son of Jesse. We had a stump of a dead tree in our backyard that began sending out shoots. Today, this former stump of a dead tree is a flourishing maple! Just so, out of the most unlikely sources (think of the prostitutes and scoundrels in David's lineage) came new life. Advent is a time of waiting and hope. With eyes of faith, watch for the bud with a heart filled with hope. Wait, like Irene in her room, for the good news.

DECEMBER 20

O Key of David

"O Key of David, O royal Power of Israel controlling at your will the gate of Heaven: Come, break down the prison walls of death for those who dwell in darkness and the shadow of death; and lead your captive people into freedom."

— *O Antiphon for Advent Vespers*

We are sitting in a corner of the big lobby — my son and his baby who is just learning to crawl. The residents in their walkers and wheelchairs stop by to chat. They are drawn by the presence of a baby. One, a slightly cranky and usually aloof gentleman, asks if he can join us in our little group. Isn't this exactly why Jesus came as a helpless infant? Who can resist a baby? Not even the grouchiest old man! A baby to unlock the hearts of the prisoners, the pagans, the wretched, the sinners.

God comes as an innocent child to open the door to heaven, to break down the prison walls of sin and death.

December 21

O Radiant Dawn

"O Radiant Dawn, splendor of eternal light, sun of justice: come, shine on those who dwell in darkness and the shadow of death."

— O Antiphon for Advent Vespers

There are those who are dwelling in the shadow of death, suffering alone, imprisoned by their illness or by their own minds. These, God holds especially close to His heart. "The light of love is born when we are touched by faith, when we open our hearts to the interior presence of the mystery" (Pope Francis, *Lumen Fidei*).

We don't always think about the fact that love is only possible because we are first loved by God, that He loved us into existence. Our minds can be darkened by our own sinfulness. We can lose sight of God's love because others have hurt us and broken our trust. So, we find ourselves seeking the face of love. And, sometimes, we are surprised when this seeking of faith meets the one whom we are seeking.

Jesus, today, shine Your light on us and on those we are caring for!

DECEMBER 22

O Keystone

"O King of all the nations, the only joy of every human heart; O Keystone of the mighty arch of man, come and save the creature you fashioned from the dust."

— *O Antiphon for Advent Vespers*

Mary wrapped the infant in swaddling clothes and laid Him in a manger. The swaddling clothes remind us of the burial shroud that would cover Jesus after His passion and death on the Cross. The manger reminds us that His body would become food for us — bread from heaven, eternal food for the soul. Christ, the keystone of the mighty arch spanning heaven and earth, became a tiny babe lying in the dust of the stable, destined to save the dust of the earth.

DECEMBER 23

God's Mystery

"Christmas invites us into this silence of God, and his mystery remains hidden to so many people because they cannot find the silence in which God acts."

— Cardinal Joseph Ratzinger, *The Blessing of Christmas*

God entered the world to bring us peace. Not to condemn the world, but to save it. And he did this by taking on our human nature, becoming a helpless baby. In this moment, we realize that money, power, and smarts are not going to save us. The helpless ones confined to their beds or stuffed away in nursing homes, the ones who are seemingly useless and powerless, these are the silent ones to whom God reveals His mystery.

DECEMBER 24

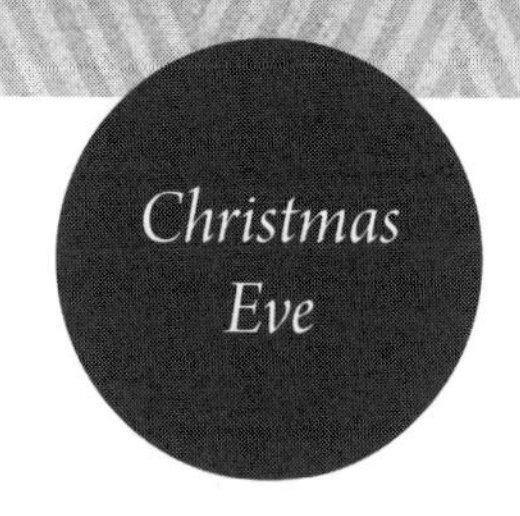

Silence

"For when peaceful stillness encompassed everything
and the night in its swift course was half spent,
Your all-powerful word from heaven's royal throne
leapt into the doomed land."

— Wisdom 18:14-15

What is the silence of God? It's not merely external silence, but a reverent silence, a space within our souls in which God's voice can be heard. Elijah heard God's voice, not in the storm or the earthquake, but as a tiny whisper, like a sigh. The clamor of the world demands our constant attention. So often our hearts have no space in which to hear God's voice.

Respect the silence. Lean your ear close to hear the whisper of the dying, the moan of the ill, or the soft breath of the sleeping infant. Sometimes, I have to simply sit with my mom and hold her hand in silence.

DECEMBER 25

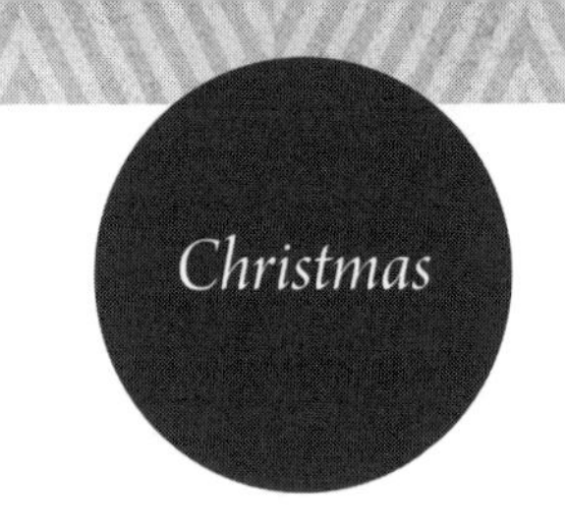

The Universal Turning Point

"The event of Bethlehem is not a romantic little idyll; it is the universal turning point, encompassing heaven and earth: God no longer remains separated from us . . . he has stepped across the dividing line to become one of us. From now on I will encounter him also in my neighbor."

— Cardinal Joseph Ratzinger, *Co-workers of the Truth*

On this day, God came to us as a little child. He came in poverty, simplicity, and helplessness, announced first to the animals and the poor shepherds. God is not like Zeus or Neptune, striking terror in our hearts in order to gain our submission. Nor is He like an earthly king who reigns amid power and splendor. Rather, He is a God who loves us. Those we care for are like the Christ Child in their simplicity, poverty, and helplessness. And perhaps that is the only path into His loving heart.

December 26

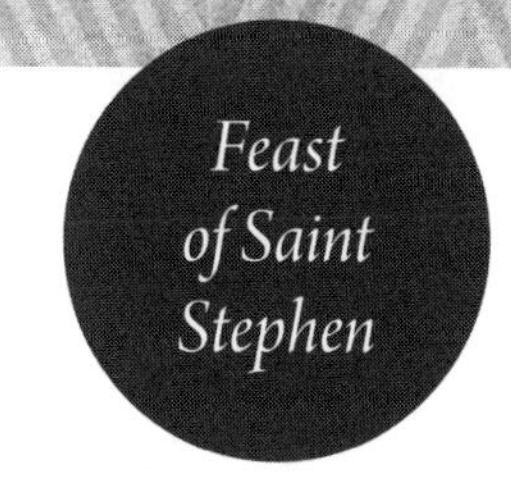

Look Up to Heaven

"Behold, I see the heavens opened and the Son of Man standing at the right hand of God."

— Acts 7:56

Just before he was stoned to death, Saint Stephen looked up and saw heaven opened. He saw the Glory of God and Jesus standing at God's right hand. Caregivers are not martyrs through the shedding of blood. Instead, you endure the "white martyrdom" of dying to yourself daily. Look up to heaven and see God smiling down on you!

DECEMBER 27

Feast of Saint John the Evangelist

At the Foot of the Cross

"When Jesus saw his mother and the disciple there whom he loved, he said to his mother, 'Woman, behold, your son.' Then he said to the disciple, 'Behold, your mother.' And from that hour the disciple took her into his home."

— John 19:26-27

John was the beloved disciple, the one whom Jesus loved. He was the one to whom Jesus entrusted the care of His mother. He was the only one of the Twelve Apostles who didn't abandon Jesus during His Passion and death on the Cross. John could do nothing to curb the crowd's vicious insults or staunch Our Lord's bloody wounds. He was helpless as Our Lord took His agonizing final breaths. Only his great love for Christ enabled him to stay throughout those long and painful hours. So, we can have confidence when we ask for Saint John's intercession. We, too, remain at the foot of our loved one's Cross.

DECEMBER 28

Feast of the Holy Innocents

Innocent Suffering

"A voice was heard in Ramah,

sobbing and loud lamentation;

Rachel weeping for her children."

— Matthew 2:18

My friend Mary's beautiful blonde daughter has never spoken. She has never been to a high school dance, never gossiped about boys. She is wheelchair-bound, mostly blind, and suffers from multiple seizures daily. She is a suffering innocent. Like the Holy Innocents who gave their lives for the Christ Child, she is holy and pure. And she blesses us with her presence, like a suffering angel in our midst.

December 29

Love Is Stronger than Death

"His kingdom is not an imaginary hereafter, situated in a future that will never arrive; his kingdom is present wherever he is loved and wherever his love reaches us."

— Pope Benedict XVI, *Spe Salvi*

You feel so helpless when your loved one is in pain. You ask God: "Why are you allowing this? Hasn't this poor one suffered enough? Where is your healing power?" And God replies, "All will be well in the end." In the end, when time ceases and "all things have taken place" (Mt 5:18), God will bring everything to His mercy and justice. We know this isn't a fairy tale,because Jesus rose from the dead. He proved definitively that love is stronger than death.

DECEMBER 30

Glory to God

"Glory to God in the highest

and on earth peace to those on whom his favor rests."

— Luke 2:14

As Pope Benedict XVI tells us, this is the very first Christmas carol — one not written by mortal men, but composed by the angels. The angels brougt the good news to the poor shepherds in the fields, keeping the night watch. Today also, God's favor rests on the poor, the humble, the sick and shut-in, the caregivers keeping the night watch. He will send His angels to give them — to give you — peace.

December 31

Kindness

"Kindness seems to know of some secret fountain of joy deep in the soul."

— Frederick William Faber, *Spiritual Conferences*

Aronnah is always smiling, laughing, eager to help. Unlike many nurses who tend to guard their positions of authority, she is always willing to do the lowlier job of a nursing assistant if the assistant is busy or having a lunch break. I ask her what she is doing for New Year's Eve, and she exclaims: "Going to church! I love to sing and pray!" I think I know the source of her ever-present kindness and joy.

"May He support us all the day long till the shades lengthen and the evening comes and the busy world is hushed and the fever of life is over and our work is done. Then in His mercy may He give us a safe lodging and a holy rest and peace at the last."

— Blessed Cardinal John Henry Newman

Acknowledgments

I wish to thank my dear and longtime friend Robin Sobrak-Seaton, who cares for her dad and her father-in-law with humor and grace, and the indomitable Mary Lenaburg (who can be found at PassionatePerseverance.blogspot.com) and her daughter Courtney. Their stories and their faith are an inspiration to me! And, of course, I wish to thank my husband, Art; and my family (Lianna, Ray, Laura, Sam, Lucy, and little Dylan) — all of whom visited my mom so lovingly and faithfully; and Cindy Cavnar, for her enthusiastic (and prayerful) support of this project. All other names in the book have been changed to protect the innocent!

About the Author

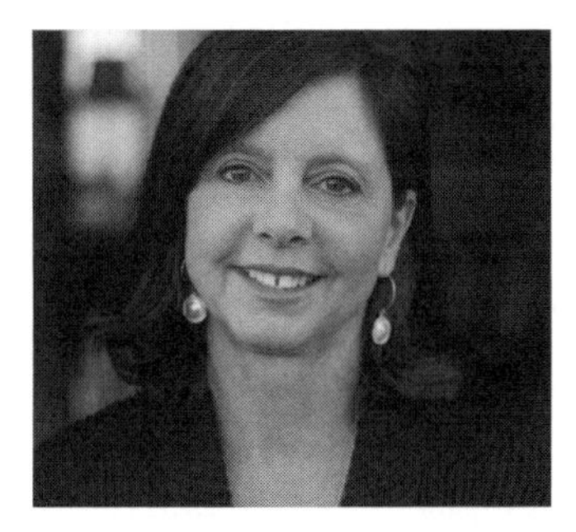

Laraine Bennett has a master's degree in philosophy and is a freelance writer for Catholic publications, including the Catholic Match Institute. She and her husband, Art, have written three books on temperament — *The Temperament God Gave You*, *The Temperament God Gave Your Spouse*, and *The Temperament God Gave Your Kids* — as well as one on emotions — *The Emotions God Gave You*.